MW00974444

0

Infectious Disease

The Guide to Residency

First edition
(This book is a reproduction of the original book "Internal medicine: The Guide to Residency" to include all the infectious disease topics with some additions)

Amer Sayed, MD
Georgia Regents University
Internal Medicine Resident

1

DISCLAIMER
Care has been taken to confirm the accuracy of the information presented in this book by reviewing the literature and books related to the subjects and by including the most common practice information and experience from the authors and editors stand of point . However, the authors, editors, and publisher are NOT responsible for errors or omissions or for any consequences from application of the information in this book and make no warranty, expressed or implied, with respect to the currency, completeness, or accuracy of the contents of the publication. Practitioners are responsible for applying this information into patient's care and the clinical out-come

The authors and editors listed the most common medicine and some of the doses used in practice according to their best knowledge, however, it is highly recommended to recheck the medicine indications and doses from an up-to-date source as they change with time. This is particularly important when the recommended agent is a new or infrequently employed drug. And it is the responsibility of the health care provider to ascertain the FDA status of each drug or device planned for use in clinical practice.

Contact the author by email: internalmedicinetheguide@gmail.com

Table of Contents

1. Antibiotics...................................14

2. Fever 25

3. White Blood Cell Count 29

4. Immune Status 34

5. Cellulitis & Osteomyelitis..........38

6. Infective endocarditis................44

7. Clostridium difficile infection.....51

8. Methicillin-Resistant
Staphylococcus Aureus 57

9. Pneumonia 61

10. Urinary tract infection.............64

12. Meningitis.................................80

13. Abdominal Pain 83

14. Medical vs Surgical Management
....89

15. Ambulatory Infections 99

16. Dermatology...........................104

17. Miscellaneous........................106

CONTRIBUTORS

All are from Georgia Regents University

Contributing Authors:
All are Georgia Regents University
Residents

Rizwan Shaikh, MD
Eduard Fatakhov, MD
Haytham Alkhaimy, MD
Scott Graupner, MD
Abhishek Mangaonkar, MD
Gita Mehta, MD
Sasha Baker, MD

Contributing Editors:
Lee A Merchen, MD, FACP
Program Director, Internal Medicine
Residency

Lu Huber, MD
Division of Nephrology
Assistant Professor

Thaddeus Carson, MD
Division of Internal Medicine
Assistant Professor

Meshia Wallace, MD
Internal Medicine Resident
Christina DeRemer, Pharm.D., BCPS
Pharmacy Supervisor, Clinical Service
(Medicine)

Mike Garcia, PhD
Director of College Composition
Assistant Professor

Medical Students:
Danielle Bayer
Brandon Taylor
Evan Fountain
Amir Makhmalbaf
Zachary Hoffmann
Reshma Reddy
Kunal Patel
Nader Aboujamous

Medical Illustrator
Michael A. Jensen, MS, CMI
Assistant Professor

Special Acknowledgement
Walter J. Moore, MD, MACP, FACR
Division of Rheumatology
Professor of Medicine and Pediatrics
**All GRU staff who provided assistance in
this project**

7

Preface

This guidebook is written to assist in the transition between medical school and internal medicine residency; it is designed to highlight the most common clinical cases presented and how best to manage them. The topics have been carefully chosen to cover common differential diagnoses to common symptoms. This book will give you a quick summary of what you need clinically to know about them as well as challenges you may encounter in the process. Ideally, this handbook can be read in 1-2 weeks and consulted at any time during residency, but especially during internship.

By reading this guide, written by current internal medicine residents, the reader will benefit from residents' actual experiences, both successes and missteps, which can aid the reader with patient care and case management. The guide includes managing the common clinical problems that patients are admitted for so the intern or the resident will feel confident and display more accuracy in examining the patient, obtaining medical history, writing a thorough and useful history and physical with appropriate work-up.

Unlike the other few available guide or pocket books, this one will NOT address unnecessary and hard-to-remember details you may NOT need in day-to-day practice in order to deliver the most high-yield information in short period of time. Since fourth-year medical students may have only one to two months of internal medicine training, they may become less familiar in managing common diseases after months of training in other specialties (NOT to mention the time traveling during match season and relocation takes). This book will prove to be efficient and effective even during this busy time.

The focus of this guide will be the common explanations for chest pain like acute coronary syndrome, pulmonary embolism; hyper/ hyponatremia, lower/ upper GI bleed, different types of pneumonia, atrial fibrillation, CHF, and so on. The primary resources and references we have used include *Harrison's Principles of Internal Medicine*, the *Washington Manual of Medical Therapeutics*, several published articles on internal medicine, and other resources. This book offers years of experience from residents and attendings,

9

keeping you, a recent medical graduate, in mind. I must reiterate that the input of the attendings who took time to be a part of this project was crucial. This finished guidebook is a culmination of real clinical experience you will encounter presented in an easy-to-reference format written by the fresh perspective and experience of your fellow internal medicine residents.

Amer Sayed, M.D.
Internal Medicine Resident
Georgia Regents University

Foreword

As has been said by many, there is no greater privilege and no more challenging responsibility than to direct the care of those who are ill. More than knowledge, it requires competency, and more than competency it requires virtue, and more than virtue it requires both passion and compassion for another human being in distress. As an internal medicine residency program director for more than 25 years, it has been my joy to observe curious, empathetic, and disciplined students develop into wonderfully compassionate and consummate clinicians. They do this by focusing fully on their patients and their wellbeing as men and women made in the Image of God, rather than data sets. Medicine is much more than making a diagnosis, prescribing a therapy, and offering a prognosis; it is a journey with another soul, sometimes for a shift, a day, a week, or decades.

Dr. Sayed's guidebook offers a convenient roadmap for the beginning of this journey. It is patient, rather than disease centered, and should be used as a starting point for the practice based learning and patient care competencies as well as virtues associated with hospital care and discharge planning. It is compact, convenient, and clear in its approach to the most common symptoms and problems of patients in modern hospitals.

Two things should be recognized by the reader, however: 1) Most hospitalized patients have more than one problem. They have multiple co-morbidities that include multiple diseases, social-economic, and especially psychological and even spiritual complexities that defy simple analysis and interact to thwart simplistic interventions. 2) Situations in which patients find themselves are always dynamic and changing, with a past which may be hidden (especially childhood trauma and abuse), a presence which needs systemic understanding, and a future which depends on timeliness and follow through of plans made.

This reference is a fine start for the genesis of an outstanding clinician. Savvy students will initiate a lifetime habit of frequent and lengthy visits to both the bedside and the enlarging greater body of literature. In each location they will ponder deeply both the causes and the effects of what is happening to their patients. Then, with experience, time, and devotion, they will be able also to taste and give to others the fruits of their practice.

12

David R. Haburchak, M.D. FACP
Professor of Medicine
Georgia Regents University

Life is short and art long, Opportunity fleeting, Experience perilous and decision difficult.

- Hippocrates

---

1. Antibiotics (abx):

The best abx choice is to send a good culture specimen for sensitivity & choose the PO form (or the IV form at first & then switch to PO as indicated) w/ consideration of the side effect, expense, frequency, & comorbidity. You can follow up the infx resolution & the abx effectiveness by monitoring the Sx, fever, ESR/CPR, WBC & clinical improvement. Know what you are treating.

Common used abx:

- **Vancomycin**: 1st line G + broad coverage, good for MRSA. IV form for broad coverage especially for sepsis or confirmed gram+ infx like strep & staph including MRSA. PO form is only for c diff infx as it does NOT absorb in GI tract. Follow up blood troughs (usually after the 3rd dose) & adjust dose accordingly (therapeutic 15-20 mcg/ml). Dosing is usually BID for normal kidney but should be changed to either daily or q48hrs for AKI or CKD stage ≥ III (pharmacy can help dosing). For ESRD patients, give the dose after the session & get trough before it as 30% will be dialyzed out. Commonly given with Zosyn as empiric therapy.

- **Clindamycin:** gram + & anaerobic, PO for anaerobic infx mainly above the diaphragm like abscess, mild cellulitis (out pt management), aspiration PNA, also effective against community MRSA (although doxycline & bactrim is better). Weak against group B strep & ↑ risk of c. diff.

- **Daptomycin**: IV, Gram positive. Usually is NOT the 1st choice & is used when Vanc fails as it has great MRSA coverage. Do NOT use for respiratory infx (pulmonary surfactant has inhibitory effect on Daptomycin, DO use in cases if osteomyelitis & skin infx. NOT classified as an aminoglycoside.

- **Zosyn (Pipercellin/Tazobactam):** IV form, 1st line broad-spectrum coverage (Gram+, - & anerobes), for moderate & severe infx like nosocomial PNA, abdomen infx (diverticulitis, abscess & peritonitis), skin infx. Does NOT cover MRSA. Can be used w/ Amikacin (aminoglycoside) to cover nosocomial pseudomonas. Commonly combined w/ Vanc as empiric Tx.

Same group: Unasyn (Ampicillin/Sulbactam), works well against G- in general (Unlike Zosyn it does NOT cover Pseudomonal species).
Augmentin (Amoxicillin/ Clavulanate) is PO & common for out-pt mild-moderate infx such as bacterial pharyngitis & sinusitis, animal bites, mild cellulitis (including diabetic foot), lower respiratory infx, & pyelonephritis.

- **Rocephin (Ceftriaxone):** IV cephalosporin, 3rd Gen, broad spectrum coverage against G+, G -, and weakly against Pseudomonas & anaerobic (do NOT use). Cephalosporins as a class of abx do NOT cover enterococcus and are not acceptable for coverage). Also doesn't cover MRSA. Use for meningitis (especially caused by S. Pneumonia or meningococcal), gonococcal infx, & prophylactic after sexual assault, UTI, skin infx, pelvic inflammatory disease, bone infx, & CAP (in combination w/ azithromycin). **Same Group: Ceftaroline:** 5th Gen cephalosporin & covers all MRSA; even Vanc resistant. **Cefdinir &**

16

Cefixime: PO 3rd G cephalosporins (good for out pt therapy)

- **Azithromycin (z pack):** common out pt PO abx for atypical PNA, bronchitis, & GPC. 5 tablets 250mg each in 1st day. 2 tabs on 1st day & then once daily. Yellow greenish phlegm does NOT automatically mean z pack. Used PO/IV for COPD exacerbation due it its anti-inflammatory effect.

- **Keflex:** 1stG cephalosporin, PO for G +. Treats bone infx, UTI, otitis media, Upper RTI, strep pharyngitis. Mainly for skin flora & surgery likes them for prophylaxis. Great for strep cellulitis infx (good for MSSA).
  Same group: Ancef & Duricef

- **Linozolid:** PO or IV, Gram + including MRSA & Enterococcus. No Gram-coverage. Usually is a 2nd line after Vanc, especially for vanc resistance enterococcus. **Treat:** CAP, HCAP & skin infx. Does NOT treat bacteremia (NOT bactericidal). Common drug interaction with SSRI = serotonin syndrome

- **Ciprofloxacin:** great for G- & pseudomonas (NOT good for G+). Used also for gastroparesis (from long standing diabetes, manifests as early satiety & N/V) to ↑ GI motility. Prolongs QT interval. Use for: UTI, GI infx, CAP. Usually orally but available IV.

Same group: Moxifloxacin & Levofloxacine (respiratory quinolones), which are preferred for CAP (good for G+ compared to Ciprofloxacin).

- **Amphotericin B:** IV, for severe fungal infx, mainly for AIDS & neutropenic /immune compromised pt w/ presumed fungal infx for empiric fungal coverage. Order fungal blood culture before initiation. Severe side effects: nephrotoxic, hydration before & while on the med. Monitor electrolytes & kidney function.

- **Fluconazole:** PO, common anti-fungal drug for either treatment of fungal infx, especially candida (oral thrush or vaginal candidiasis) & severe cases like cryptococcal meningitis in AIDS, or prophylaxis in immunosuppressed pts like in BMT. High doses can treat fungemia. Diflucan 150mg one dose po is a common Tx for vaginal candidiasis w/ white cheesy discharge (Vaginal

Miconazole is another option). **Nystatin** is good for Candida infx like vaginal w/ creamy discharge, PO w/ white painful lesions or thrush, & skin candida (or Tenia) w/ white flaky red skin w/ itching (use w/ combination of steroid like **Betamethasone** for Symptomatic relief).

Clotrimazole topical is also effective against candida & most of other topical fungal infx (including athlete foot).

Same group: Voriconazole (good for mold like Aspergillus as fluconazole does NOT cover mold) & **Itraconazole**: for presumed serious fungal infx (comes in PO form).

- **Metronidazole (Flagyl):** below diaphragm anaerobes, 1st choice for clostridium difficile infx, vaginal infx (vaginosis w/ thin fishy smelling discharge & trichomoniasis w/ greenish yellowish discharge), Colorecatal infx, Giardia & Amebia infx (anaerobes) . Category B in pregnancy (A accepted, D life threatening). Avoid Alcohol & educate about metallic taste.
- **Amikacin:** Aminoglycoside IV covers G- mainly. Treat: UTI, meningitis (G-

infx), HCAP including Pseudomonas respiratory infx. Renal & neurologic side effects and also ototoxic.

Same group: Gentamycin & Tobramycin (the best for pseudomonas & G-)

- **Doripenem:** broad coverage (GPC, GNB, & anerobic) except MRSA. Included in carbapenem class of abx. Good for pseudomonas (ventilator-associated PNA or VAP). Only IV & is NOT usually 1st line Tx. Usually switched to it from zosyn if it fails for possible resistance (greater gram negative coverage).

Same group: Meropenem carries↑ risk of seizure in pt w/ CNS issues & **Ertapenem**, which is NOT covering pseudomonas but still good broad coverage (used once daily IV).

- **Aztreonam (monobactam abx):** IV/IM broad coverage for G- including *Pseudomonas aeruginosa* (NOT good for G+ or anerobic). It is a synthetic monocyclic beta-lactam antibiotic (amonobactam). It is usually NOT the first line & used when other agents fail covering G- infx (like for UTI). Alternative agent in penicillin allergy (low cross reactivity).

- **Bactrim:** Sulfa drug, usually PO. Very common use: PCP infx (& prophylactically) in immunosuppressed pts, UTI (lower for 3 days & upper use IV or PO for extended duration ~14days), skin & soft tissue infx, CA-MRSA, & COPD exacerbation. Caution w/ sulfa allergy & in pregnancy (category C).
- **Acyclovir:** effective against Herpes Zoster infx (shingles) if administered within 72 hrs from onset of blistering to reduce pain & ↓ duration. Another indication: herpetic encephalitis & genital herpes. Hydrate well before & during Tx due to risk of AKI. Same group: **ganciclovir** (mainly for CMV infx)

Special considerations:

- **Good culture specimens**
  - **Sputum:** Squamous epithelial cells line the mouth. If> 10 of these cells are present in the specimen then it is may be sputum w/ saliva but if<10 per hpf & >25 PMNs in the specimen, it is more likely to be from the lungs.

Consider bronchoscopy by pulmonology for good sputum samples if needed.

o **Urine:** mid-stream clean catch (foley cath is NOT a good sample as it is may be colonized w/ bacteria).

o **Abscess:** the wall of the cavity & NOT the pus (which is WBC & debris & may NOT have bacteria growing).

o **Osteomyelitis:** Cx curettage from the ulcer base following superficial debridement of necrotic tissue. Organisms cultured from superficial swabs are NOT reliable for predicting the pathogens responsible for deeper infx. Bone biopsy & Cx is important before initiating therapy especially in chronic osteomyelitis.

> **Attention!** Findings that indicate failing regimen and require switching abx for possible resistance include: 1. persistent fever after 48-72 hours, 2. clinical deterioration 3. worsening erythema (ex. cellulitis beyond initially marked borders).

- **MRSA abx:** Vancomycin, Daptomycin & Linezolid (for hospital acquired MRSA) & Doxcycyline, Bactrim, Rifampin & Clinamycin (for community acquired MRSA).
- **Pseudomonas abx:** Zosyn, cipro/Levofloxacin, Cefepime, Ceftazidime, Mero/Imi/Doripenem (Ertapenem is NOT good for Pseudomonas), Topramycin/Gentamycin/Amikacine, Aztreonam, Fosfomycin, & Colistin
- **Same bioavailability if they are given IV or PO:** Azithromycin, Levofloxacin, Ciprofloxacin, doxycycline, clindamycin, linezolid, & fluconazole.
- **You can choose either IV or PO abx** depending on the specific infx you are treating. Endocarditis may need IV abx for 6 weeks (PICC line will be

useful) but treating something like PNA or UTI→ it's ok to start IV & switch to PO or even begin w/ PO. PO intolerance makes IV route a good option. For bacteremia start IV & check for one negative blood Cx. After 2-3 days switch to PO if negative.

- **Antimicrobial stewardship program** (program for wise abx use) De-escalation of therapy, IV to PO conversions, Dose optimization, Guidelines & clinical pathways, Education (Colonization vs. infx). Implementation of an antimicrobial stewardship program helps: Improve pt outcomes, Improve pt safety, Reduce resistance, & Reduce cost.

2. Fever

A normal temperature is 37°C & variation of +/- 1 degree is normal (low grade fever is 37.5-38.0). Medically significant fever is >38 (or 100. 4 F).

H & P:
Exposure to infected person, chills, sweating, fatigue, rash, dehydration, or ↓ appetite. The degree of fever does NOT necessarily reflect the severity of the infx. Although infx is the most common reason for fever, consider other reasons such as cancer, infarction, CNS disease (e.g. hemorrhage), clot, recent procedures (e.g. bronchoscopy), & meds.

Management
- **Tests:** CBC w/ differential (elevated WBC, & bandemia/left shift indicated infx), ESR & CRP, urine analysis, CXR, pan-culture (urine, blood & sputum) as indicated.
- **Tx:** Empiric abx (e.g. Vanc & Zosyn) can be started on pts w/ comorbidities (e.g. ESRD, CHF, COPD, cancer, etc.) after sending the cultures. You can stop abx if there are no indications of infx from the tests, or

resume them if the source of infx found (de-escalate the abx depending on the sensitivity results). Consider meningitis & infective endocarditis (especially in pts w/ prosthetic valves) because a missed diagnosis can be catastrophic.

Special considerations:

- Elderly pts, pts w/ chronic hepatic or renal failure, & pts taking glucocorticoids may have **infx w/o fever.** A hypothermia may be an indication of infx in this subset of pts.
- Although subjective fevers need to be considered, **use objective measurements** for accurate assessment.
- **Check the absolute neutrophil count** because neutropenic fever is an emergency (start broad spectrum abx after obtaining pan-cultures (order a CXR & urine analysis as indicated).
- **Rash** (or skin erythema/abnormality) should be evaluated in febrile pts. Broad differential including but not limited to bacterial infx [ex. Rickettsia & Lyme disease - tick borne illnesses, meningococcus, cellulitis or

osteomyelitis (NOT typically rash but erythema)] & viral infx such as mononucleosis (EBV/CMV).

- **Antipyretics** (acetaminophen & NSAIDs) can be given for fever. They do NOT cause harm & do NOT slow the resolution of common viral & bacterial infx. However, w/ bacterial infx, withholding antipyretic therapy can be helpful in evaluating the effectiveness of a particular abx, particularly in the absence of positive cultures of the infecting organism. Cold compressors/ice packs can reduce fever as well.
- **Consider quick tests** like the Streptococcus test, influenza A/B swab as indicated to start abx or Tamiflu, respectively (effective in the first 24-48 of onset of signs & symptoms). Also consider respiratory pathogens panel.

> **Attention**: Do NOT culture more than once w/ in 24 hrs for pts who spike fevers (in case of an unidentified source of infx).

- **Daily reassessment** of abx regimen should we done to determine if they are still indicated & whether the symptoms (like fever) are still present. Consider adding antifungal or antiviral meds for immunocompromised pts who are still febrile on empiric antibacterial coverage.
- **Postoperative fever** is common & etiology usually coincide with post-op day:
  - Day 1-2 – atelectasis (use incentive spirometry) & HCAP
  - Day 3-4 – Foley associated UTI, catheter - related blood stream infx, wonder drug
  - Day 5 - surgical site infx
  - Day 7 - DVT or simply normal from the inflammation/stress of the surgery (or 5Ws: wind, water, wonderdrug, wound, walk)

3. White Blood Cell Count

Quick facts regarding interpretation of WBC results, which are encountered on a daily basis in the inpatient setting:

- **Elevated WBC count** (normal 4. 5-10k) is usually an indication of infx, especially if there are bands in the differential. Normal percentage is 3-5% and bands>8% indicates infx. Bands reflect a "left shift" which is an ↑ in the number of immature leukocytes due to body's rapid effort in mounting a stronger immune response.
- **Immune status should be assessed** for every the individual pt, as the infx may present differently in immunocompromised pts (cancer, chemotherapy, steroids, HIV, transplant etc.) versus immunocompetent (fever can be the only presenting Sx).
- Erythema/swelling for localized infx & elevated WBC may be absent due to the weak immune response. Abx coverage & prophylactic measures are different depending on the

immune status (consider CD4 count or absolute neutrophil count).

- **Fever, sweat, fatigue, elevated ESR & CRP along w/ elevated WBC** are all indications for infx & immune response. The source of infx is important to identify (URI, UTI, abscess, PNA, meningitis, etc.), & the history & physical can give clues to the source. In addition consider ordering pan-cultures w/ sensitivity (blood, urine, & sputum), UA, CXR, or lumbar puncture depending on the hx.

- **Neutrophil percentage is elevated mostly from a bacterial infx** (70% is normal) **& lymphocytes from viral/fungal infx** (20% is normal).

- **An elevated WBC is NOT always from infx:** although it is the most common reason. Steroid use, cancer, infarction, stress, recent procedure, anemia, burn, & pregnancy are also other causes of elevated WBC count that must be taken into account, especially if there are no other signs of infx.

- **A ↓ WBC count, <4K, can be a sign of infx as well,** especially in elderly pts, who no longer mount a functional immune response. It is also one of the

SIRS criteria which dictates when medical intervention is indicated.

- **Neutropenic fever** is an emergency. Oral temperature is greater than 38.3°C & the absolute neutrophil count (ANC) is less than 500. Hospital admission & starting broad-spectrum IV abx are warranted, including possibly Vanc, Zosyn, & fluconazole. Most of the neutropenic pts w/ fever are cancer or post-chemotherapy pts.

> **Attention**: Neupogen (filgrastim) is a granulocyte colony stimulating factor that can be used to ↑ WBC count post-chemotherapy if indicated. In most cases, it is used per Hem/Onc recommendations (no role in acute infx).

- **Often times, a very ↑ WBC count, >50K,** is assumed to be from leukemia/lymphoma, such as CML. However, ↑ WBC count can be caused by a leukemoid reaction from an infx, NOT malignancy, and usually returns to normal when infx is treated.

- **Excessive IV fluids** can cause a dilution effect leading to a ↓ in all blood cell lines, including WBCs
- WBC count can be followed w/ a CBC on a daily basis to monitor the effectiveness of an abxTx. If it is still elevated after 1-2 days of initiating empiric abx, this may indicate a need to adjust abx.
- **Common WBC abnormal values:**
  1) **Spontaneous benign peritonitis** (SBP) WBC >250 (in peritoneal fluid). Peritoneal dialysis (PD) fluid WBC >100 is indication of infx.
  2) **CSF** normal WBC 0-5, bacterial meningitis WBC>500, viral WBC>100
  3) **Arthrocentesis:** synovial fluid WBC>50K in bacterial/septic joint while in crystal inflammation (like gout) can be up to 10-20K (synovial fluid microscopy & culture is needed)
  4) **WBC>10 in urinalysis** is pyuria, one of the signs of UTI (normally <5 & absence of leukocyte esterase)
- **Abnormal WBC (>12K or <4K) is 1 out of 4 SIRS criteria.** SIRS can be diagnosed in the presence of 2 or more of the following (notice that hypotension is NOT part of SIRS criteria):

1. ↑ temperature (>38. 3 or <36)
2. Tachypnea (RR >20)
2. Tachycardia (HR >90)
3. WBC count >12K or <4K or >10% bands

4. Immune Status

Immune-compromised pts need special attention because they do NOT have the ability to respond normally to an infx due to an impaired or weakened immune system. This inability to fight infx can be caused by a number of conditions including diseases (eg. diabetes, HIV, uremia), malnutrition, sickle cell disease, asplenia, chronic abx, elderly, ESRD on dialysis, malignancy, & drugs (chronic steroids, immune-suppressive/transplant & immune-modulating meds).

- **Assess immune status for all the pts**, especially if their presenting condition is infectious (diagnoses & abx option are different depending on immune status).

Attention: unusual opportunistic infx like fungi (candida & cryptococcus), viruses (CMP, HSV & PK), & certain bacteria may NOT cause persistent infx in normal people. Signs of infx may NOT be as prominent in the immune-competent pts.

- High-grade fever, elevated WBC w/ left shift, pain & guarding (in intra-abdominal infx), nuchal rigidity (in meningitis), & dysuria (in UTI) may NOT all be present in infx. High suspicion of infx & starting empiric abx coverage after obtaining the appropriate tests & cultures is essential & possibly even life-saving.

> **Attention:** Non-specific findings like loss of appetite, fatigue, N/V, & hypotension and tachycardia (amongst other signs of shock) put infection high on the differential.

Special considerations

- Most pts w/ immunodeficiency can safely receive all killed or inactivated **vaccines**. In contrast, live vaccines should NOT be given to pts w/ severe immune dysfunction.
- **Prophylactic abx** are indicated in pts w/ specific immunodeficiency disorders in order to prevent opportunistic infx: Diflucan for fungus, Bactrim for PCP infx (prophylactic dose every 48h), acyclovir.
- **PCP prophylaxis in non HIV pts:** Pts receiving a glucocorticoid dose equivalent to ≥20 mg of prednisone

daily for at least one month can also be considered immune-compromise [i.e. transplant pts (bone marrow or solid organs like kidney); pts receiving certain immunosuppressive drugs (purine analog or another T-cell depleting agent). Generally the need for prophylaxis is NOT permanent; however, it depends on the indication. HIV/AIDS pts w/ CD4 count <200 may need Bactrim until their CD4 count ↑

- **Neutropenic fever:** a single PO temperature of >38. 3°C (101°F) or a temperature of >38. 0°C (100. 4°F) sustained for >1 hr (NOT just subjective fever) in pts w/ absolute neutrophil count (ANB) <500. There are many etiologies for neutropenia, but some of the most common are recent chemotherapy & acute leukemia. Cover prophylactically w/ empiric parenteral abx therapy (such as vanc/zosyn), fluconazole, & acyclovir after sending pan cultures (blood/urine/sputum), & proceed w/ the work-up as indicated (CXR & urine analysis- UA). Neutropenic fever is a medical emergency & empiric antibacterial therapy should be started w/ in 60 minutes of presentation in all pts.

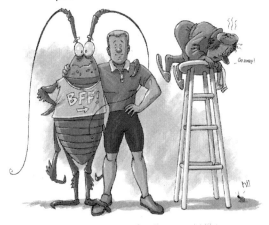

Immunocompromised pts manifest infx & get treated differently than immunocompetent.

5. Cellulitis & Osteomyelitis

- **Cellulitis** is an infx of the skin & subcutaneous tissue. Manifest as erythema (rubor), warmth (calor), pain (dolor), & edema (tumor), in the absence of underlying suppurative foci (such as an abscess which needs additional I & D). Lymphangitis (proximal red streaking) & lymphadenopathy may be present.
- **Predisposing factors include:** disruption of skin barrier w/ trauma, as well as edema (venous insufficiency or CHF). Most commonly caused by beta-hemolytic Strep & Staph, including MRSA. Gram-negative bacilli are common in diabetic & immunocompromised pts Staph infx tend to be associated w/ abscess formation.
- **Diagnosis** is clinical & blood cx positive in few. Aspirate of bulla or pus from furuncle or pustule may provide diagnoses & culture sensitivity to narrow down the choice of abx. Mark the affected skin w/ a pen to monitor progression.

- **Treatment** involves abx either PO for mild cases (ex. augmentin, clindamycin, or cephalexin) or IV if systemic toxicity is present (empiric Tx w/ Vanc & Zosyn). Vanc is effective against MRSA. Doxycycline alone is also effective against MRSA & Strep for out pt. Re-evaluate the affected area & treat the underlying predisposing conditions (ex. DM or lower extremities edema).

Special considerations

- **DDx:** necrotizing fasciitis (crepitus on physical exam & subcutaneous air on x-ray), gas gangrene (crepitus on exam), toxic shock syndrome, osteomyelitis, skin abscess (fluctuation & need surgical drainage), herpes zoster (vesicles in dermatomal distribution), DVT (usually unilateral, warm, hx of immobility, especially after orthopedic procedures; Tx: anticoagx for 3-6 months if 1st time), venous insufficiency (bilateral, chronic, standing for long periods of time, no systemic sx), crystal inflammation such as gout or pseudogout (usually 1st metatarsal, may show monosodium urate crystals from joint aspirate).

- **Necrotizing fasciitis** is a deep infx of the subcutaneous tissue that results in progressive destruction of fascia & fat. The affected area is usually erythematous (w/o sharp margins), swollen, warm, shiny, & exquisitely tender. There can be fulminant tissue destruction w/ systemic signs of toxicity, resulting in ↑ mortality rates. Associated conditions include diabetes, substance abuse, obesity, immunosuppression, recent surgery, & traumatic wounds. Caused by either polymicrobial or Group A Strep. **Tx:** first start w/ broad-spectrum empiric abx therapy & hemodynamic support and early aggressive surgical exploration & debridement of necrotic tissue.

- **Pts w/ lower extremities edema** may benefit from Tx w/ compressive stockings & diuretic therapy to prevent recurrent cellulitis.

- **Special cellulitis:** Cat bites (*P. multocida*); dog bites (*P. multocida, C. canimorsus*); human bites (*E. corrodens*); penetrating injury like

nails (*Pseudomonas*);
gardening injury (*Sporothrix*).
- **IV abx** can be started for few days & then switched to PO if pt is improving.

> **Attention**: Skin flora, like Strep & Staph, are still the most common causes of the cellulitis after the bite injury (treated w/ Vanc for in pt & clindamycin or Bactrim for out pt). Vaccination status for tetanus & rabies should be determined and treated accordingly.

Acute Osteomyelitis:
- Infx of bone due to hematogenous seeding (S. aureus) or direct spread from contiguous focus from skin damage from trauma (S. aureus & S. epidermidis). Local findings such as erythema, warmth, swelling, & pain may be present along w/ systemic signs such as fever, night sweats, & malaise.
- **Management:** Identification of the causative organism is key. Blood cultures & needle bx or surgical sampling. Radiologic work up: X-ray (needs time to be abnormal), MRI (detects early changes) & bone scan

($\downarrow$ specificity as it will be positive in cellulitis as well). Tx: Abx (based on Cx data) for 4-6 weeks. WBC count, ESR & CRP are significantly elevated & they can be monitored if abx resistance is a concern. ID & orthopedic surgery may need to be consulted.

Chronic osteomyelitis
- **Management:** May NOT see leukocytosis. Identify the causative organism (by a surgical biopsy/ culture before starting abx) & start abx according to C & S. Consider surgery evaluation for acute osteomyelitis that fails to respond to medical therapy, chronic osteomyelitis, complications of pyogenic vertebral osteomyelitis (e.g., early signs of cord compression, spinal instability, epidural abscess), & infected prosthesis. Best evaluated by X-ray & MRI.

Diabetic foot: infected neuropathic foot ulcer. Usually is complicated w/ arterial impairment. Tx: bed rest, elevation, non–weight-bearing status, wound care, abx. For mild or out pt, use Augmentin or Cephalexin.

Add Bactrim if MRSA is suspected. For severe or in pt: Vanc & Zosyn (or Imipenem) for 6 weeks.

6. Infective endocarditis

Infx of the endocardium manifested by the prototypical lesion, vegetation, and most commonly located on heart valves. Consider it in case of Bacteremia (mostly w/ gram + cocci as they "stick" to the heart valves unlike gram -bacillus), fever of unknown origin, new onset heart failure, acute weight loss & pts w/ risk factors like prosthetic valves (bio or mechanical).

- **Etiology:** Typical organisms causing endocarditis are: Staphylococcus aureus (commonly associated w/ intravascular devices & injection drug abuse), Streptococci (group B & viridans group), HACEK group (Hemophilus, Actinobacillus, Cardiobacterium, Eikenella & Kingella). Prosthetic valve endocarditis is most often associated w/ S. aureus, coagulase negative staph, enterococci, gram-negative bacilli, viridans strep & Candida SP.

- **Types:** Endocarditis is typically classified into *acute, subacute, & prosthetic valve endocarditis.* Acute endocarditis typically presents over 5 to 10 days & is often associated w/

Staphylococcus aureus & gram-negative bacilli (less common). Subacute endocarditis typically presents over weeks to months & is associated w/ Streptococcus species.

- **Clinical features:** Fever, chills, sweats, anorexia, weight loss, malaise, myalgia and/or arthralgia, back pain, new or changing heart murmurs, splenomegaly, clubbing, Osler's nodes, Janeway lesions, subungual hemorrhages, Roth's spots, petechiae, neurologic manifestations.
- **Work-up:** Positive blood cultures & demonstration of vegetation(s) on an echocardiogram are two major criteria for diagnosis (see below for criteria). Other lab abnormalities which are seen in IE are anemia, leukocytosis, hematuria, elevated ESR, CRP, RF, ↓ serum complement.
- **Clinical diagnosis-** *Duke Criteria* are often used:

Major criteria	Minor criteria
Positive blood culture: Typical microorganism from 2 separate blood cultures, OR For atypical microorganisms, persistently positive blood cultures (blood cultures drawn 12 hrs apart or all of the 3 sets of blood cultures or majority of 4 separate blood cultures are positive, w/ 1st & last culture drawn >1hr apart), OR Single positive blood culture of Coxiellaburnetii or phase I IgG antibody titer of >1: 800. **Evidence of endocardial involvement:**	1. **Predisposing heart condition or IVDA** 2. **Fever** >38 C 3. **Vascular phenomena** (Arterial emboli, septic emboli, mycotic aneurysm, intracranial hemorrhage, conjunctival hemorrhage, Janeway lesions). 4. **Immunologic phenomena** (glomerulonephritis, Osler's nodes, Roth's spots, rheumatoid factor). 5. **Microbiologic evidence:** + blood culture but NOT meeting

Positive echocardiogram: Oscillating intra-cardiac mass on valve or supporting structures, **OR** Abscess, **OR** New partial dehiscence of prosthetic valve, **OR** New valvular regurgitation.	major criteria or serologic evidence of active infx w/ typical microorganism.

- For diagnosis, 2 major OR 1 major & 3 minor OR 5 minor criteria are essential.

Please note
- TTE is accurate in only about 65% cases of endocarditis. Hence, if clinical suspicion is high, always order a TEE, which is accurate in >90% cases.
- When endocarditis is very likely, a negative TEE does NOT exclude diagnosis & should be repeated in 7-10 days.
- TEE is the optimal method for diagnosis of prosthetic valve endocarditis or detection of myocardial abscess, valve perforation or intra-cardiac fistula.

- Follow-up TEE or TTE is needed to re-assess vegetations, complications, or Tx response.

Management
IV abx for extended periods of time (usually for 6 weeks, consider PICC line). Start w/ broad empiric Tx like Vanc & Zosyn (G+ coverage is essential) & then narrow down depends on susceptibility (usually ID are involved).

Endocarditis prophylaxis
1. Prophylaxis is recommended for the following conditions:
   a. Prosthetic valves.
   b. Previous endocarditis.
   c. Unrepaired congenital heart disease, including palliative shunts or conduits.
   d. Repaired congenital heart disease w/ prosthetic material during 1st 6 months of procedure
   e. Cardiac valvulopathy in transplant recipients.
2. Dental, PO or respiratory tract procedures require prophylaxis in the above-mentioned conditions.
3. GI & genitourinary procedures DO NOT require routine prophylaxis;

however, high-risk pts infected or colonized w/ enterococci should receive amoxicillin, ampicillin or Vanc prior to urinary tract manipulation.
4. Prophylaxis is recommended for procedures on infected skin, skin structures or musculoskeletal tissue for conditions mentioned above.
5. Prophylaxis is w/ amoxicillin or ampicillin 30 minutes to 1 hour before procedure (clindamycin, cephalexin, azithromycin, clarithromycin, or clindamycin if penicillin allergic).

Special considerations
- In general, consider infective endocarditis if you have sick pts with more than one damaged organs at the same time w/o good explanation like new onset CHF & AKI (from valvular disease from the vegetations & from septic embolism)
- Streptococcus gallolyticus (previously known as Streptococcus bovis) is associated w/ colon polyps & tumors.

Attention: G- organisms bacteremia usually does NOT cause IE (no need for TEE unless you have very high suspicion) while G+ organisms does (sticky organisms).

- Unusual form of endocarditis resulting from endocardial damage due to abnormal blood flow is NBTE (non-bacterial thrombotic endocarditis); seen commonly in valvular abnormalities such as mitral & aortic regurgitation, ventricular septal defect & congenital heart defects. When uninfected vegetations occur in malignancy, chronic diseases, Systemic Lupus Erythematosus (SLE) & anti-phospholipid syndrome, it is known as marantic endocarditis.

7. Clostridium difficile infection (CDI)

C. difficile infx is a major cause of inpatient gastrointestinal illness. C. difficile is a gram-positive, spore-forming, normal flora of the GI tract mostly spread by the fecal-oral route. Soap & water is the best for prophylaxis (alcohol foam does NOT eliminate spores).

- **Risk factors:** Recent abx use is the main culprit, especially clindamycin, cephalosporins, & fluoroquinolones. Though, any abx can predispose to *C. difficile* overgrowth, including Vanc & metronidazole. Nursing home pts, elderly, immunosuppressed, & pts w/ altered GI anatomy (e.g., ileostomy, colostomy) are at ↑ risk.
- **Clinical features:** Typical presentation is profuse watery diarrhea, lower abdominal pain/tenderness, & often extremely foul-smelling stool (nurses usually suspect that first).
- **Laboratory tests:** The most accurate test is stool *C. difficile* antigen PCR. The disadvantage is that it takes around 24-48 hrs to return from the

lab. Get CBC & CMP to assess severity.

- **Classification:** Used to decide on Tx options, including possible escalation to ICU level of care.
    - ○ **Mild:** Diarrhea is the sole Sx.
    - ○ **Moderate:** Diarrhea plus additional signs & Sx NOT meeting criteria for severe or complicated CDI.
    - ○ **Severe:** Hypoalbuminemia (albumin <3), a WBC count >15 k, & abdominal tenderness. **Complicated CDI pts who need to be considered for ICU:** HoTN w/ or w/o vasopressors, fever > 38. 5°C, ileus, abdominal distension, mental status changes, WBC count >35, 000or <2, 000, serum lactate level >2. 2 mmol/L, & any signs of end-organ failure.
- **Treatment:** Can be initiated before laboratory confirmation for pts w/ a ↑ pre-test suspicion. STOP the offending abx. If abx must be continued, treat w/ abx less known for causing CDI, such as

aminoglycosides, macrolides, Vanc, or tetracycline.

- **Mild-to-moderate**: PO metronidazole 500mg TID x10 days should be used. If the pt fails to respond to metronidazole therapy, a change in therapy to PO Vanc should be considered.
- **Severe or complicated disease:**
- **w/o ileus** → PO Vanc is administered (in addition to IV metronidazole)
- **w/ ileus** →Vanc delivered PO & per rectum plus IV metronidazole is to be given. Additionally, supportive care w/ fluid resuscitation, electrolyte replacement, & DVT prophylaxis should be continued. A CT abdomen & pelvis is recommended in pts w/ complicated CDI, as is a surgical consult due to possible need for subtotal colectomy & ileostomy, which is associated w/ ↓ mortality.
- **Recurrent disease**: The **first recurrence** of CDI should be

treated w/ the same regimen used for the initial episode. However, if infx is severe, PO Vanc should be used. The **second recurrence** should be treated w/ Vanc PO. For a **third recurrence** after a pulsed Vanc regimen, fecal microbiota transplant (FMT) should be considered.

Special considerations:

- **Fidaxomicin** - approved for mild-to-moderate CDI & was non-inferior to Vanc in phase III trials & **Fecal microbiol transplant (FMT)** has shown promising results in trials for recurrent CDI as mentioned above.

> **Attention**: Probiotics are NOT recommended according to current guidelines, especially in immunosuppressed pts, where there are a few case reports of bacteremia resulting from their use.

- **PO Vanc is expensive;** PO metronidazole is cheap.

- **Do NOT test C. diff in pts w/o diarrhea** (unless you have another reason like leukocytosis w/o known source). Monitor response to Tx by ↓ bowel movement numbers per day. Recovery is monitored clinically (usually no need to test negative C. diff as it can be positive after the Tx for months w/o the need to repeat abx & it is NOT a sign of Tx failure).
- **Not all inpts with diarrhea have CDI, consider broader workup.**
- **Start counting 14 days of anti C diff abx (like Flagyl or Vanc) from the time you stop the offending agent** (like Clindamycin). Do NOT undertreat in order to avoid recurrence.

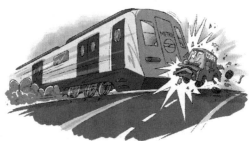

METROnidazole is effective against C diff infx.

8. Methicillin-Resistant Staphylococcus Aureus (MRSA)

This is a major cause of morbidity & mortality in hospitals. It can cause PNA, bacteremia, and skin &skin structure infx (SSSIs). Tx has become challenging because of resistance & limited availability of antimicrobial agents. Moreover, there has been an emergence of community-acquired strains (CA-MRSA), which sometimes have a higher virulence than hospital-acquired ones.

- **Community-acquired MRSA:** Clindamycin, trimethoprim-sulfamethoxazole (TMP-SMX) & tetracyclines (doxycycline) are recommended as first line agents for CA-MRSA, but should NOT be used for hospital-acquired strains due to ↑ resistance. Out of the 3 agents mentioned above, only clindamycin has good activity against both MRSA & beta-hemolytic Streptococci. Usually, in skin infx thought to be due to MRSA, empiric coverage for both MRSA & Streptococci is needed. However, using clindamycin as a sole agent can lead to resistance. Hence, TMP-SMX or doxycycline in combination w/ a beta-lactam agent, such as ampicillin or amoxicillin, is preferred.

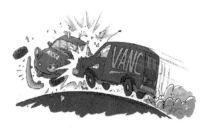

*VANcomycin is the 1st empiric IV Tx of choice for **MRSA**; especially for in pt.*

> **Attention**: Clindamycin is associated w/ a relatively higher risk for *c diff infx*.

- **Hospital-acquired MRSA:** Nursing homes, dialysis centers, or any long-term healthcare facility. IV Vanc is cheap, effective, & has years of data proving 1st line efficacy. However, in recent years, there have been reports

- of ↑ resistance & rising minimum inhibitory concentrations (MICs).
- There are reports of emergence of VRSA (Vanc resistant *S. aureus*), VISA (Vanc intermediate *S. aureus*), & HVRSA (heterogeneous Vanc resistant *S. aureus*). **Currently** it is still used as a 1st line agent.
- Vanc is bactericidal via inhibition of cell wall synthesis. Only used IV formulation (unless specifically treating *C. difficile* infx). **Requires dose adjustment in renal insufficiency.** Nephrotoxicity requires stopping the drug. Red man syndrome (flushing & itching) requires pretreatment with antihistamine & slow infusion. Trough (blood level) should be checked regularly to assure therapeutic levels (obtain true trough by checking before 4th dose or before HD).
- **Linezolid** can be used in both PO & IV formulations (equal bioavailability). It has good lung penetration & is recommended for MRSA PNA NOT responding well to Vanc & inpts being discharged back to a nursing home on PO meds.

- **Daptomycin** is used for MRSA bacteremia, NOT recommended for use in MRSA PNA (inactivated by pulm surfactant). Can be used for complicated skin infx & infective endocarditis. Adverse effects include myopathy (monitor CPK), peripheral neuropathy, & eosinophilic PNA.
- **Ceftaroline** **(Cephalosporin)** approved for PNA & cellulitis (NOT 1st line therapy)

9. Pneumonia (PNA)

PNA is a very common cause for hospital admissions. Knowing how to appropriately recognize & treat PNA is an essential part of internal medicine.

- **Signs & symptoms:** Fever, cough, yellow-greenish sputum (in **both** bacterial & viral infx), pleuritic CP, dyspnea, & tachypnea
- **Work-up:** Hx, vitals, physical exam (crackles on auscultation, egophony, tactile fremitus), CXR (infiltration & opacities sometimes are hard to notice & differentiate them from atelectasia), sputum/blood cultures, Strep urine antigen, CBC w/ differential, BMP, & other labs as pertinent (legionella antigen, fungal cultures, respiratory panel, LDH); pleural thoracentesis & bronchoscopy (BAL) if indicated.

Pneumonia Types & Management
- **Community Acquired Pneumonia (CAP):** Pneumonia acquired outside of medical facility that does NOT fit in the definition of HCAP. Standard out pt therapy is monotherapy w/ a fluoroquinolone (Levaquin) or

Augmentin + Azithromycin. In hospital setting, start Ceftriaxone/Azithromycin IV.

- **Healthcare Associated Pneumonia (HCAP):** Criteria include hospitalization in acute care hospital for two or more days in last 90 days, residence in nursing home or long-term care facility in last 30 days, receiving out pt IV therapy or home wound care in last 30 days, or attending hospital clinic or dialysis center w/ in 30 days. Also included PNA that begins 48-72 hrs after hospital admission. Standard abx are Vanc & Zosyn IV (covers G+, G-, & anaerobic including MRSA & Pseudomonas) as initial therapy. Tailor therapy according to C & S.
- **Ventilator Associated Pneumonia (VAP):** PNA occurring after 48 hrs of pt being intubated & placed on mechanical ventilation. Tx is same as for HCAP (must cover Pseudomonas).

Special considerations
- **Community Acquired PNA Risk Stratification:** good standard guide for admission is **CURB-65:** Confusion, Uremia (BUN >20), Respiratory rate >30, Blood pressure <90/60, Age >65.

Score of 0-1: out pt. Score of 2: in pt. Score of 3 or greater: assess for ICU.

- **There are many types of PNA**: bacterial, viral (self-limited/supportive management/Tamiflu within 1st 48hrs of symptom onset), fungal (certain places & immunocompromised pts) causes but this is a good guide for initial management.

- **PNA can be hard to diagnose clinically** for some pts especially CHF pts (BNP may help) & more testing is needed (CXR or chest CT scan). Atelectasis on CXR can look similar to infiltration, which is THE objective sign in PNA diagnosis. Correlate w/ the clinical picture & do NOT feel obligated to a full course of abx if PNA was misdiagnosed.

> **Attention:** Repeat CXR in 12-24hrs (for comparison) as PNA infiltration unlikely to resolve but atelectasis or fluid edema may do (especially if diuresis is given).

10. Urinary tract infection (UTI)

Generally categorized into either upper or lower UTI. Lower UTI Sx: dysuria, ↑ frequency, urgency, hematuria & suprapubic pain while upper UTI (or pyelonephritis) Sx: fevers, chills, sweats, N/V, vomiting, diarrhea, & flank or abdominal pain. Lower UTI Sx may also precede these Sx.

Another way to categorize UTIs:
- **Uncomplicated** – affects the 1st lower UTI for female
- **Complicated** -affects the rest (like any upper UTI for either sex, any UTI in male, recurrent lower UTI in female).

Urine analysis (UA) is an easy, cheap & fast diagnostic test for UTI (although Sx & physical exam can be enough). Elevated WBC, esterase (sign of WBC), nitrates (sign of bacteria) & RBC (±) presence along w/ bacteria is positive in any UTI. Leukocytosis & bandemia along w/ positive blood culture can be found in upper UTI.

Management:

Uncomplicated UTI: You can start the empiric Tx based only on the Sx.
- **In non-pregnant female:** 3 days of TMP-SMX, 5 days of Nitrofurantoin or single dose (3 grams) of Fosfomycin
- **In pregnant female:** Ampicillin, Fosfomycin, Nitrofurantoin, Keflex, Aztreonam or Cefixime for 7-10 days (longer than usual). Repeat urine Cx to assure resolution in a monthly bases & Tx even asymptomatic bacteriuria in pregnancy as they are high risk for frank UTI (30-40%) due to progesterone effect as a smooth muscle relaxant.

Complicated UTI: Obtain urine culture then initiate Tx empirically for 7-14 days w/ Ciprofloxacin PO or IV (be aware of QT prolongation & get a baseline EKG, consider another abx if QT is already prolonged or pt is on other QT prolonging meds like haldol).

Upper UTI (pyelonephritis):
- **For young pts who can tolerate PO intake & are relatively**

healthy: consider PO fluoroquinolone like Ciprofloxacin for 7 to 14 days (you may NOT need urine analysis or urine culture). Consider hospital admission & IV Ciprofloxacin if the pt has N/V & then discharge on PO Ciprofloxacin when PO is tolerated.

- **Choose broad-spectrum coverage w/ extended-spectrum beta lactam like zosyn or carbapenem in the following settings:** suspected resistant organism (like recurrent UTI & indwelling foley cath), recent abx use, urinary obstruction & immunosuppression. You can add gram positive coverage like Vanc in case of septic shock or complicated pts (like elderly w/ multiple comorbidities)

- **Obtain Renal Ultrasound or CT** for persistent fevers or continuing Sx after 72 hrs of abx to evaluate for complications of pyelonephrosis (e.g., perinephric abscess).

- **Obtain Urine culture** especially for hospitalized pts & de-escalate (or optimize) abx if empiric agents like Zosyn/vanc were started

Special consideration:

- **Pts w/ chronic Foley catheter** may always have UA positive for WBC, esterase & bacteria which is due to colonization; so do NOT treat unless Sx are present (elevated blood WBC, fever, dysuria or any systemic infx signs).

> **Attention**: UTI is a common reason for AMS or GI Sx like N/V in elderly; so do NOT forget to check UA in elderly.

- **Treat asymptomatic bacteriuria** (positive bacteria in UA w/ no WBC or esterase) only in pregnant women & prior to invasive urologic procedure. Some pts w/ chronic indwelling Foley like spinal injury pt, or prostate cancer pts, as well as ESRD pts on HD can have positive UA (+ bacteria, nitrate & esterase) but Tx w/ abx is NOT indicated unless they are Symptomatic (fever, dysuria, elevated WBC, or sepsis). Usually the bacteria in this case are very resistant & strong abx like imipramine should be reserved for a later time when the pt is in real need (eg: septic shock or Sx)

- **Upper UTI is a common cause of sepsis or septic shock** (which can be informally called Urosepsis) & it should be highly considered in septic pts even w/o urinary Sx, especially for elderly w/ altered mental status. IV abx should be initiated w/ in 1 hr along w/ stat IV hydration (follow sepsis protocol)

- **Foley catheter should be discontinued as soon as it is NOT indicated** due to an↑ risk of iatrogenic (preventable) UTI. Consider condom cath (still ↑ UTI risk x2 comparing to no cath at all but is still better than foley cath) or urinal to get accurate ins & outs as indicated.

- **UTI diagnosis can be challenging sometime:** for septic patients (w/ AMS & unknown dysuria hx) with mildly positive UA (like negative nitrate, weak + esterase, 5 WBC & +1 bacteria). In critical pts → empirically treat w/ abx while you pan-culture & look for another source of infx.

11. Shock & Sepsis

Survival of the critically ill pt depends on initiating life-saving measures in a timely fashion. However, recognizing serious illness before the onset of overt instability can be challenging. For example, younger pts w/ sepsis can appear deceptively well but may develop multiorgan failure w/ in hrs. A systematic approach to pt assessment minimizes the likelihood of delayed recognition of critical illness.

The initial evaluation should consist of a brief bedside hx & focused examination to discern whether immediate action is needed to stabilize the pt's airway, breathing, or circulation. Review of vital signs over the preceding hrs often provides valuable information on the pt's overall current stability.

Common early interventions include intravenous fluid boluses for HoTN, O_2 & noninvasive ventilatory support for respiratory distress, & naloxone or dextrose (D50) for encephalopathy due to narcotics & hypoglycemia, respectively. Studies that may be useful for diagnosing the cause &

determining severity of illness include ABG; CBG, Hgb, lactic acid levels, EKG, & portable CXR. Limited bedside TTE to assess the hemodynamic status of unstable pts has ↑ in recent years (i.e.: IVC compressibility).

After imminently life-threatening issues are addressed, a **more comprehensive secondary assessment** should be performed w/ an emphasis on identifying less obvious evidence of organ hypoperfusion. This includes AMS (confusion, agitation), ↓ urine output (<0.5cc/kg/hr), skin changes (pallor, diaphoresis, cyanosis, cool extremities), & ↑ work of breathing.

Shock is a state of ↓ tissue perfusion (mostly from HoTN), which can result in inadequate O_2 delivery for cellular needs (tissue ischemia). Tissues ischemia often results in organ dysfunction if severe or prolonged (usually >30 minutes).

Signs for shock: systolic BP <90, MAP<60, signs of end organ damage from hypoperfusion (↓ urine output, AMS, CP, lactic acidosis from the anaerobic metabolism) & lack of BP response after IV fluid challenge (usually after 2-3 Liters boluses).

Three main types of shock:
1. **Cardiogenic** (massive MI or pulm embolism),
2. **Septic** (from severe infx or anaphylaxis)
3. **Hypovolemic** (severe dehydration or bleeding).

Blood Pressure = Cardiac Output (Heart Rate x Stroke Volume) x Resistance

BP is consistent of few parameters including: peripheral resistance (mainly ↓ in septic shock), cardiac output (mainly ↓ in cardiogenic shock like in MI or CHF but also can be ↓ in septic shock du to the negative cardiac effect from the septic toxins) & preload or blood volume (mainly ↓ in bleeding/ dehydration & even in septic shock → hypovolemia occur due to ↑ capillary permeability & 3rd space loss).

In all types of shock, the therapeutic goals are to support tissues & organs that are dysfunctional or at risk of damage due to hypoperfusion & to restore perfusion if possible.

Perfusion can often be improved by administering some combination of intravenous fluids, vasopressors/ inotropic agents such as:

- **Norepinephrine (levophed):** which is strong α1 agonist (stronger than epinephrine) & β1 agonist (same as Epi)/ moderate β2 agonist (weaker than Epi). "Squeeze" good but **proarrhythmic due to β1 effect**.

> **Attention:** β2 agonist causes HoTN (receptors are in vessels) vs β1 agonist ↑ chronotropic and inotropic effect (receptors in the heart) vs α1 agonist in vessels (NOT in the heart) →

- **Phenylephrine:** which is strong α1 agonist. "Squeeze" good but do NOT affect the heart.
- **Vasopressin:** which is a V1 receptor agonist in the vascular smooth muscle of the vessels. Also "squeeze" w/o cardiac direct effect).
- **Dopamine & dobutamine:** less common
- **Epinephrine:** β agonist mainly

Understanding the cause of shock & reversing the cause of the abnormal physiologic parameter is the key to successful outcomes. Such directed Tx could include lysis of a massive pulm embolism causing cardiogenic shock or Tx of an infx causing septic shock. If ↑ fluid volume is likely to improve perfusion, intravenous fluids should be given liberally as boluses w/ immediate clinical reassessment (septic pts may need up to 6 liters in the 1st 6 hrs). The adoption of guidelines using physiologic parameters, such as central venous pressure, as targets for resuscitation has improved outcomes by encouraging more timely administration of needed fluids (mostly used is normal saline).

> **Attention**: the adaption of guidelines using physiologic parameters, such as central venous pressure CVP, as targets for resuscitation has improved outcomes by encouraging more timely administration of needed fluids (mostly used is

Aggressive volume expansion is most important in pts w/ hypovolemic shock & has also been associated w/ improved outcomes in pts w/ septic shock. Concern about precipitating heart failure & pulm edema

72

should NOT modify the need for large bolus volume administration (intubate if needed).

Sepsis
Sepsis is an exaggerated inflammatory response to an infectious stimulus & is characterized by a severe catabolic reaction, widespread endothelial dysfunction, & release of inflammatory agents. The mortality rate of pts w/ sepsis complicated by multiorgan failure may be greater than 70% to 90%; mortality rate can be estimated by adding 15% to 20% predicted mortality for each sepsis-induced organ dysfunction. The term/s:

- **Systemic inflammatory response syndrome (SIRS)** was introduced to describe findings of:
  1. Altered temperature (<36 or >38)
  2. Tachycardia (>100)
  3. Hyperventilation (>20)
  4. Abnormal WBC (<4, 000 or >12, 000) regardless of the cause (inflammatory or infectious).
- **Sepsis** is defined as SIRS plus suspected (or proven) infx (UTI, PNA, cellulitis, etc.).
- **Severe sepsis** is associated w/ systemic effects including: HoTN, ↓ urine output, or metabolic acidosis.

73

- **Septic shock** is sepsis w/ persistent organ hypoperfusion despite adequate initial fluid resuscitation, which is usually 30cc/kg (like 3 liters for 100kg pt. That requires vasopressor agents to maintain blood pressure).

> **Attention**: Septic shock requires persistant HoTN (NOT responsive to IV fluid) but sepsis can

Management
Treat infx (empiric abx like vanc/zosyn w/ in 30 minutes of recognizing sepsis, if possible) & optimize tissue perfusion (by aggressive fluid resuscitation & vasopressors). Repetitive fluid challenges are performed by giving a 500 to 1000 mL bolus of crystalloid over short intervals while assessing response to target central venous pressure (normal is 8-10, higher number is may be better in case of septic shock).

Most pts need 4 to 6 L of fluid in the first 6 hrs, & a frequent error is underestimating the intravascular volume deficit & the amount of fluid required. Use of crystalloid or colloid is likely equivalent. Vasopressor therapy should be started immediately if the initial fluid challenge fails to restore adequate blood pressure & organ perfusion.

Prolonged hypoperfusion results in worsening ischemia & organ failure. Vasopressor therapy w/ norepinephrine, vasopressin, or phenylephrine is frequently needed to restore perfusion during life-threatening HoTN.

No trials have established a single superior vasopressor agent. Norepinephrine, vasopressor, phenylephrine are 1st-line agents for correcting HoTN in septic shock. Vasopressor agents can be used concurrently w/ fluid resuscitation in life-threatening HoTN.

Being at the upper side of fluid resuscitation is better than under resuscitation & intubate prn if pulm edema & CHF is a concern. Get lactic acid q4-6hrs & monitor the trend; down trending is reassuring & up trending may indicate plan/intervention changing.

Special considerations:

- **Assess the need for lines** such as arterial line, central line, hemodialysis line, Foley cath.

Attention: short line (like peripheral large lines) are better for resuscitation than long/ narrow lines (like PICC/ central lines) due to ↑ fluid flow resistance with ↑ line length and ↓ line radius.

- **Consider prophylactic meds** like GI ulcers w/ PPI & DVT w/ heparin SQ & check for decubitus ulcers in all ICU pts.
- **Low-dose corticosteroids** as indicated in septic shock refractory to fluids & vasopressor therapy
- **Bicarbonate should NOT be used** for the purpose of improving hemodynamics or reducing vasopressor requirement when treating lactic acidosis w/ a pH higher than 7.15.
- **Always consider:** avoiding malnutrition, employing therapist-driven weaning protocols, using sedation protocols w/ a daily interruption in ventilated pts, using intermittent or bolus sedation rather than continuous infusions, & avoiding neuromuscular blockade as possible.

- **Code blue:** ACLS algorithm (**available online**).
  As a quick review:
  1. Unresponsive?
  2. Pulseless?
  3. Start chest compression
  4. IV access/heart rhythm? (Place monitor pads) /intubation?
  5. Consider Electrical cardioversion (VF, VTach, or SVT?), IV meds (epi/HCO_3/Mag/IV fluid/amio) prn
  6. Send for basic blood work (CBG, CBC, CMP, lactate, troponin, D Dimer, ABG, etc)
  7. Check the chart, nurse, or primary team for any possible etiology, recent meds or intervention could be related to the code (like high insulin dose or new meds).

Assess pulse & heart rhythm q2min → check BP if you had *Return Of Spontaneous Circulation* (*ROSC*) & transfer to ICU. Attempt to call family to update them.

Do not do chest compression on an "awake person".

12. Meningitis

Telltale symptoms are fever & neck stiffness usually present with or without altered mental status. Onset can be abrupt. Generalized HA radiating to the neck that is constant & severe. **Bacterial Meningitis is a medical emergency!**

- Aggravated by flexion of the neck - **Brudzinski's sign** (flexing the neck causes flexion of the hips & knees); **Kernig's sign** (pain w/ flexing the hip at 90° & then trying to fully extend the knee; high false positive rate)

- **Diagnosed** w/ urgent LP with CSF gram stain & treated w/ urgent IV abx if **bacterial** (CSF: low glucose -0.4 of blood glucose-, high protein & WBC ->500-w/ neutrophil predominance). **Tx:** Vanc + Rocephin IV); Symptomatic Tx if **viral** (WBC -<300- w/ lymph

> **Attention**: "Partially treated meningitis" is when the pt gets abx before the LP and CSF may not (elevated WBC & protein and low glucose). Consider abx until CSF culture is negative.

- predominance, mild protein elevation & normal glucose). Consider **Steroids** in bacterial meningitis & get ID help if available.
- Always obtain blood cultures and if possible get a head CT prior to performing LP (if your patient has an intact immune system head CT isn't required).
- Post-neurosurgery or patients with head trauma should be covered with vancomycin & ceftazidime or cefepime
- Dexamethasone prior to or shortly after initial abx for 4 days reduces poor neurologic outcomes in bacterial meningitis patients specifically affected by Pneumococcus.
- Aseptic meningitis occurs after URI or pharyngitis caused by viruses and drugs (Bactrim or NSAIDs). LP will have lymphocytic pleocytosis. Obtain viral PCR of

> **Attention**: In pregnant & immune compromised patients broad spectrum of abx to treat for *Listeria monocytogenes* with Ampicillin or penicillin-G. If penicillin allergic use Bactrim.

likely culprits (i.e. HSV, enteroviruses, HIV).

13. Abdominal Pain

Abdominal pain is Sx that the vast majority of people will experience sometime in their life, & it has multiple causes.

History
- **Rule out the presence of the surgical abdomen** as this can kill the pt quickly. Make sure that the pt is hemodynamically stable.
- **Timing:** acute vs. chronic; gradual vs. sudden
- **Location**: localized vs. referred pain
- **Quality**: sharp, dull, tearing, burning, & boring; has the quality changed over time?
- **Prior episodes** of similar pain, relationship to **menstrual** cycles (female)
- **Associated Sx**: N/V, diarrhea, constipation, fever, etc.
- **Previous intra-abdominal procedures** such as appendectomy, cholecystectomy, & laparoscopies. Be concerned for small bowel obstruction secondary to adhesions.
- **Last bowel movement:** time & quality (soft or hard), this important as

Attention: flatulence is reassuring as it complete rules out Small Bowel Obstruction (SBO)!

constipation can cause abdominal pain.

- **Exacerbating or relieving** factors such as food, bowel movements, & deep breathe, positional, etc.
- **Presence of fresh blood** (hematochezia) vs. old blood (melena)

Physical exam
- Assess for any signs of an inferior MI as angina may present as epigastric pain
- Check for localized tenderness, rebound, guarding, & bowel sounds
- Stool guaiac PRN (but no need to perform FOBT if pt has frank blood because you already have your answer)
- Any woman of child bearing age who complains of lower abdominal/pelvic pain should get a pelvic examination
- **Murphy's sign:** pain on palpation of the right subcostal area during inspiration/p**cholecystitis**
- **Psoas or obturator sign:** pain upon passive extension of the thigh w/ knees extended while the pt is lying on their side → **appendicitis.**

- Rectal exam (should NOT be performed on neutropenic pts)
- **Carnett test:** used to distinguish intra-abdominal pain from abdominal wall pain. Press in the location of the pain & have the pt do a sit-up. If the pain worsens w/ the sit-up→ the pain is from the abdominal wall
- Pain that is out of proportion to the abdominal exam is suggestive of acute **mesenteric ischemia** (usually PMHx of CVA, CAD, PAD, or erectile dysfunction ED).
- Immunosuppressed pts may have benign exam despite a surgical abdomen.

Labs
- CBC, chemistry panel, liver function tests, amylase & lipase, lactate, coagulation panel
- Type & cross (if surgical abdomen or blood in stool)
- Urinalysis & urine pregnancy test
- In a pt w/ ascites that is having new abdominal pain or fever- a paracentesis must be performed to r/o SBP (spontaneous bacterial peritonitis). SBP is present if neutrophil count in the fluid is >250.

Abdominal pain: differential by pain location

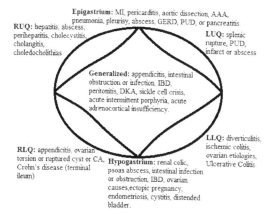

Epigastrium: MI, pericarditis, aortic dissection, AAA, pneumonia, pleurisy, abscess, GERD, PUD, or pancreatitis

RUQ: hepatitis, abscess, perihepatitis, cholecystitis, cholangitis, choledocholithias

LUQ: splenic rupture, PUD, infarct or abscess

Generalized: appendicitis, intestinal obstruction or infection, IBD, peritonitis, DKA, sickle cell crisis, acute intermittent porphyria, acute adrenocortical insufficiency.

RLQ: appendicitis, ovarian torsion or ruptured cyst or CA, Crohn's disease (terminal ileum)

Hypogastrium: renal colic, psoas abscess, intestinal infection or obstruction, IBD, ovarian causes, ectopic pregnancy, endometriosis, cystitis, distended bladder.

LLQ: diverticulitis, ischemic colitis, ovarian etiologies, Ulcerative Colitis

Radiology

- **Abdominal series:** r/o the presence of free air under the diaphragm, obstruction, volvulus, sentinel loop, toxic megacolon (> 7 cm in mid-transverse colon diameter), pleural effusion (pleurisy, pancreatitis if effusion is left-sided), etc.
- **Ultrasound:** to investigate hepatobiliary pathology if RUQ pain

- **CT abdomen/pelvis:** to r/o diverticular disease, appendicitis, & colitis
- Other studies will depend on the pt's specific situation

Management
- **If there is potential for a surgical abdomen, request a surgical consultation** & keep the pt NPO. Consider IV hydration. Type & cross for packed RBCs. Watch for septic/hypovolemic shock. Hang appropriate abx (like Ciprofloxacin & flagyl for GI infx source) early if there is suspicion for ascending cholangitis, diverticulitis, sepsis, etc.
- Try a **GI cocktail (**30 ml of Mylanta or Maalox + 10 ml of viscous lidocaine ± 10 ml of Donnatal) if dyspepsia is a possibility
- **Consider starting a PPI drip** if pt w/ active GI bleed, & consult GI along w/ getting Hgb & hematocrit (H & H) Q6hr
- **Partial SBO** (usually from previous surgery adhesions) is managed conservatively by bowel rest w/ NG tube, IV fluid & pain management.

14. Medical vs Surgical Management

This is a very important topic, & most likely this will be life-saving if the pt is appropriately triaged to the correct service. Most of these pts will be evaluated in the Emergency room, & sometimes the pt can develop complications on the floor, especially in our oncology population. Therefore, this topic will address key diseases where early diagnosis for medical or surgical management is critical. Don't forget just because the abdominal pain is NOT pronounced, does NOT mean it is NOT life threatening. Always think about the surgical options for treating any medical case & know when they can help.

Pancreatitis: Diagnosed w/ elevated lipase (more specific) & amylase (more sensitive). Always perform the Modified Ranson's criteria on admission & at 48 hrs (**available online**) to estimate mortality. Most common causes are EtOH & gallstones (worse), as well as, elevated triglyceride or Ca. If concerned for diagnosis is unclear or you want to r/o necrotizing pancreatitis→ obtain CT scan abdomen, which is NOT necessary for diagnoses. Surgical management along w/ GI consultation is always merited in cases of worsening necrotizing pancreatitis or unresolved pseudocysts (usually after wall cysts maturation, if possible).

> **Attention:** Amylase and lipase are useful in only making pancreatitis diagnosis (>3 times elevation of normal limits). However it does not indicate the severity of the pancreatitis and should NOT be followed for monitoring the pt improvement or worsening.

Medical management of acute or acute on chronic pancreatitis is appropriate w/ mild disease, which subsides in a few days. The pancreas is given rest, w/ I. V. Fluids. Ringer's Lactate is now the preferred fluid of choice in all pancreatitis pts. Morphine or meperidine should be given for pain control. Avoid TPN at all cases, even in severe pancreatitis. Instead, a post pyloric feeding tube (NJ tube) may be placed. Continue the clear liquid diet until diet can be advanced to regular diet (advance diet as soon as tolerated) when abdominal pain improves. If pancreatitis is caused due to biliary obstructions then, laparoscopic cholecystectomy might be performed during the in pt hospital stay.

Diverticulitis: is inflammation or infx of the diverticular pouches w/ fecal impaction that can lead to erosion & bowel perforation.

Management:

- Do **CT scan** to identify pts who are likely to respond to conservative medical therapy or will need surgery evaluation.
  Conservative Tx (Bowel rest w/ NPO or/& NJ tube & abx) in pts w/ uncomplicated diverticulitis → success rate is 70 – 100%.
- Decide **Out pt vs. In pt** based on severity of presentation, the ability to tolerate PO intake, the presence of comorbid diseases, & the available support system need to be taken into account. Hospitalization is required for immunosuppressed, the elderly, those w/ significant comorbidities, & those w/ ↑ fever or significant leukocytosis.

- **Abx:**
  In pt ABX: Average 10 – 14 days depending on resolution of Sx. Gram-negative rods & anaerobes (particularly *E. coli* & *Bacteroides fragilis*) are the usual causes of diverticulitis: Fluoroquinolones w/ metronidazole, Amoxicillin-clavulanate, or TMP-SMX w/ metronidazole are the options.
  Out pt: 10 – 14 day of Ciprofloxacin & metronidazole. Ciprofloxacin is the best option because it has better coverage of gram-negative pathogens. **Another option** is Amoxicillin-clavulanate. If NOT tolerable to metronidazole use Clindamycin/moxifloxacin.
- 6 weeks after recovery pts should undergo a colonoscopy to exclude other diagnosis. Considerations such as colonic neoplasia & to evaluate the extent of the diverticulosis.
- **Surgery Indications:**
  Absolute **indication**: Complications of diverticulitis (peritonitis, abscess, fistula, obstruction), clinical deterioration or failure to improve w/ medical

therapy, recurrent episodes, intractable Sx (sepsis), or inability to exclude carcinoma. Recurrence diverticulitis rate is 35%

- **Surgical goals:** remove the septic focus by resection of the colon, treat obstruction or fistula, & restore bowel continuity (while minimizing morbidity & mortality).

- **Laparoscopic vs. open resection:** Laparoscopic surgeries are associated w/ a shorter recovery time. Fast-track recovery protocols improve perioperative outcomes in pts for whom elective laparoscopic surgery is performed. Shorter time to consuming a soft diet (2. 3 vs. 3. 6 days), 1st bowel movement (2. 6 vs. 3. 5 days), median length of hospital stay (3 vs. 5 days), & lower morbidity (15 vs. 26%) compared w/ pts managed w/ traditional postoperative care.

Cholelithiasis: (gallstone) is a concentration of crystalline product formed in the gallbladder by bile components. These calculi may pass distally into other parts of the biliary tract & cause obstruction, which leads to cholecystitis. These pts usually present w/ complaints of biliary colic & postprandial (particularly w/ fatty foods) right upper quadrant pain lasting a few hrs.

- **Medical Tx:** mostly out pt, but can prescribe ursodeoxycholic acid (Ursodiol) therapy 300 mg BID for long-term management & pain control w/ NSAIDs. If the pt is experiencing recurrent cholelithiasis then elective cholecystectomy can be performed to prevent future attacks of biliary colic.

- **Acute cholecystitis:** occurs most commonly due to obstruction. Pts may present acutely w/ RUQ pain, fever, leukocytosis, ↑ levels of ALK-P & GGT. Right upper quadrant ultrasound showing a thickened gallbladder wall & /or stones is diagnostic. Empiric abx (vanc/zosyn) should be started promptly on admission & given prior to surgery. Surgery is usually recommended w/ in the first 3 days of admission. In ↑ risk pts, or the ones who are too sick or unstable to undergo surgery, a percutaneous drainage device should be placed by Interventional Radiology along w/ abxTx.

- **Acute Cholangitis:** is a biliary tract infx, usually caused by an infx building behind a stone obstruction. The pt presents w/ a triad of Sx: Fever + Jaundice + RUQ pain = Charcot's triad. If you add AMS + HoTN + Charcot's Triad = Reynolds's Pentad. Pt should have GI medicine along w/ surgery consult, & will most likely need ERCP & removal of the stone.

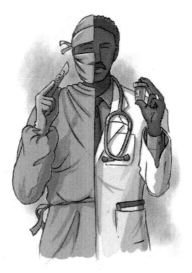

Surgery & Medicine are complementary & needed to ensure the best pt outcomes.

Special consideration:
- **Hold strong pain meds to assess abdominal pain** progression so you do NOT miss catastrophic surgical event (in equivocal cases)

- **Septic knee effusion (septic joint) needs immediate arthrocentesis** to prevent long-term joint damage & help w/ diagnoses. Do NOT forget NPO if you suspect surgery or you have a pt w/ N/V & suspect bowel obstruction (consider NG tube).
- **Bowel ischemia** needs high suspicion & may need an emergent surgery consult to evaluate for bowel resection if it's NOT viable to prevent sepsis, f/u w/ lactic acid.
- **Trending Lactic acid** is helpful in case of any suspected ischemia (indicator of anaerobic metabolism). Reassuring if it is trending down
- **Empyema (pus in pleura, seen on chest ct scan) or abscess (in general)** needs drainage along w/ medical management. Pancreatitis & pancreatic cysts afterwards are commonly medically managed even if the necrotic tissue is up to 30% & surgery indication is very limited (in case of infected necrosis from CT scan guided FNA sample).
- **Other cases you can ask for surgical help when indicated:** Chronic osteomyelitis (ask vascular surgery to evaluate for amputation

when perfusion is poor & refractory to abx), urinary obstruction (urology evaluation for nephrostomy in case of AKI), Pericardial effusion (for CT surgery evaluation in case of tamponade suspicion), spinal cord compression (Neurosurgery)

- **Pt's wishes are important to know** in case they do NOT want surgery so you can start/continue medical management ASAP
- **Assess the ability of lying flat:** for any surgical procedure as the anesthesia & surgery team will need to know that (CHF & COPD pts may NOT be able to lay flat &, therefore, will need different approaches)
- **Always get INR/PT/PTT/platelets count before any invasive procedure** or surgery to assess bleeding risk. Make sure pt is NPO at least 6-8 hrs before. ASA usually is fine to resume but in neurosurgery procedures. Plavix needs to be held for at least 5 days (to wash off).

15. Ambulatory Infections

- **URI:** presents w/ cough (with green/yellow sputum which does NOT necessarily means bacterial infx but could be viral), fever, & dyspnea. Viral mostly associated w/ headache, runny nose, sneezing, conjunctivitis, sick contact & pt does NOT look very sick (viral is self-

---

Attention: **CENTOR criteria** can guide to start abx (mainly used for pharyngitis); as it is hard to differentiate between viral vs bacterial infx by just physical exam or radiology.

Ask about 4 things: 1. Fever >38 C, 2. Cervical adenopathy, 3. Tonsillar exudates, & the absent of cough or rhinitis (calculator available online).
0-1: no abx
2-3: rapid strep swab test & if positive→ start abx (z pack or Augmentin),
4: start abx w/o further testing.

---

limited & treat supportively w/ 1st G antihistamine, cough suppressant, and other symptomatic medications). If bacterial: Azithromycin (z pack) is a good option.

- **Pharyngitis**: sore throat, tonsillar exudates, cervical lymphadenopathy, *absence of cough.* Most cases self-limited & don't require abx. Usually viral but group A beta-hemolytic strept is common culprit which is diagnosed by rapid-strept test. **Treatment is required for those susceptible to rheumatic fever**. 1st obtain culture, then start pen V, clindamycin, or azithromycin (Z-pak)

- **Sinusitis**: nasal discharge, headache, facial tenderness, tooth pain. Acute infx is usually viral, bacterial culprits: *pneumococcus, H. influenza, M. catarrhalis.* If symptoms persist > 10 days think anaerobes. Chronic infx > 12 weeks of mucopurulent drainage, nasal obstruction, facial pain/pressure, decreased olfaction. Predisposing factors: asthma, nasal polyps, allergies, or immunodeficiency Dx: plain films NOT recommended, objective evidence of mucosal discharge via rhinoscopy or nasal endoscopy with cultures. Symptomatic: oral decongestants, analgesics, +/- topical decongestants or intranasal steroids. Abx: if symptoms persist for > 10 days or symptom management fails start with 5-7 days of augmentin or doxycycline or respiratory quinolone if penicillin allergic.

- **Influenza**: outbreaks usually in winter months of febrile illness with headache, myalgia, cough, and malaise. Dx is usually clinical, can be confirmed with nasopharyngeal swab. Treatment usually supportive with focus on hydration and analgesia. If patient presents within 24-48 hours of symptom onset antiviral medication has been proven to shorten duration of illness. Oseltamivir or zanamivir for 5 days has been used to treat and provide prophylaxis for influenza A & B. Amantadine and rimantadine are only affective against influenza A.

- **Acute Bronchitis**: cough +/- sputum, chest discomfort, and SOB lasting from 1-2 weeks with or without fever caused by bronchial inflammation from virus or bacteria. Diagnosis is clinical and treatment is usually supportive with cough suppressants. If symptoms last > 2 weeks consider pertussis and obtain nasopharyngeal swab and treat with z-pak.

UTI: see chapter 10. If lower (suprapubic tenderness, dysuria, frequency) order urine analysis & start abx (like bactrim or Ciprofloxacin for 3 days if uncomplicated), if upper UTI (fever, chills, CVA tenderness, dysuria) order UA & assess the need for hospital admission (elderly, multiple comorbidities, septic signs, etc) for IV abx (Ciprofloxacin or zosyn). UTI can be categorized to "uncomplicated", which is in lower UTI in female for the 1st time. The rest is complicated (male even for the 1st time, recurrence, Upper UTI, etc).

Attention: no need to follow UTI response to abx by urine analysis or urine Cx. Clinical improvement is enough (unless in pregnancy → Tx even asymptomatic bacteriuria and assure resolution w/ negative urine Cx)

---

16. Dermatology

- **Shingles:** Reactivation of latent varicella-zoster virus (VZV) infx w/ in the sensory ganglia results in herpes zoster or "shingles". This syndrome is usually characterized by a painful, unilateral vesicular eruption in a dermatomal distribution. Early antiviral therapy (acyclovir for 1 week for age >50) can promote rapid healing of skin lesions, lessen the severity & duration of pain associated w/ acute neuritis, & reduces the incidence or severity of chronic pain. Post herpetic neuralgia is a common sequelae after initial infection resovles. Tx: gabapentin or pregabalin (early acyclovir helps ↓ duration & ↓severity)

- **Tinea or dermatophytes** are superficial fungal infections that are routinely diagnosed by location, scraping lesions and using KOH prep to visualize the fungus. **Body** –tinea corporus, pink ring shape & rx topical azole, **Scalp**- tinea capitus, areas of scaling +/- hair loss/itching, rx oral antifungal, **Nail**-

tinea unguium (onychomycosis) thickening and opacification of nail rx oral antifungal, **Foot-** tinea pedis, scaling, redness, and itching/burning, rx topical antifungal, keep feet dry and teach proper hygiene, **Groin/thigh** – tinea cruris, scaling & redness usually sparing scrotum, rx topical antifungal & keep area dry, teach proper hygiene

- **Scabies**: is another possible itching etiology, which usually presents w/ severe itching, often worse at night, & nondescript erythematous papules. Family involvement strongly suggests the diagnosis. **Tx:** Ivermectine PO (which can treat lice too) & /or Permethrin (Tx the family also & wash the linens).

17. Miscellaneous

- Gastroenteritis: presents w/ nausea & vomiting usually. Etiology is mostly viral (self-limiting) and Tx is hydration PO (IV if severe dehydration, PO intolerance, AKI, comorbities or elderly). Antibiotics (azithromycine PO) is good for traveler's diarrhea, high fever (suspect bacterial etiology), severe abd pain, prolonged diarrhea, resent hospitalization/ abx use (check C. dif), bloody stool (NO abx for E coli O157 →↑ risk HUS). Anti-diarrhea meds (like Imodium) is good for severe diarrhea (can NOT adequately replacing fluid), especially if not bacterial (do NOT keep bacteria in GI system by anti-diarrhea). Immune compromised pts can have different etiologies like: Cryptococcus, CMV or MAC (will need more comprehensive testing). Testing like stool Cx, parasites/ oval, stool WBC, C. diff, or stool lactoferrin are warranted in specific cases

(alarming Sx: severe abd pain, bloody, high fever, severe dehydration)

- **HIV:** fairly common, anti-retroviral therapy ARVT are usually initiated by ID doctors and usually they interact w/ most of the other medicine (check interaction when you start any new meds). For example: Pravastatin is maybe better than Lipitor for CAD pts as the later has severe interaction w/ protease inhibitor. Always check CD4 (<400 →AIDS), prophylactic meds (Bactrim DS every other day for PCP, Azithromycine for MAC), opportunistic infx, atypical presentations for infx (no fever, no nuchal rigidity for meningitis,.etc)

- **Tuberculosis:** can present in many ways and needs high suspicion to diagnose. Screening for pre-employment exam, immigrants, health care professionals by PPD and then chest x-ray (if PPD+) to look for an active lesions is very common. Blood QuantiFERON gold is a faster alternative to screen high risk pts.

Vaccines:
    Influenza: yearly for all adults.
    Pneumonia vaccines (Pneumovax): pneumococcal polysaccharide vaccine (PPSV23), elderly>65, DM, CHF, CKD, Asthma/COPD, asplenic pts, & others.

> **Attention**: Usually screening tests are NOT recommended for pt >75 yo or pts w/ life expectancy <10 years (physician dependent).

    Zoster: > 60 yo, one time (life attenuated).
    Other life attenuated vaccines: Varicella, MMR, yellow fever, oral polio, & Nasal flu (most of the others are inactivated).
    Tdap/Td: >19 yo, one time (but tetanus q10 yrs)
    HPV vaccine: all male & female age 13-26 yo.

Reference:

1. Tomasz A. Antibiotic resistance in Streptococcus pneumoniae. Clin Infect Dis 1997; 24 Suppl 1:S85.
2. Mulligan ME, Murray-Leisure KA, Ribner BS, et al. Methicillin-resistant Staphylococcus aureus: a consensus review of the microbiology, pathogenesis, and epidemiology with implications for prevention and management. Am J Med 1993; 94:313.
3. Jacobson KL, Cohen SH, Inciardi JF, et al. The relationship between antecedent antibiotic use and resistance to extended-spectrum cephalosporins in group I beta-lactamase-producing organisms. Clin Infect Dis 1995; 21:1107.
4. Tamma PD, Girdwood SC, Gopaul R, et al. The use of cefepime for treating AmpC β-lactamase-producing Enterobacteriaceae. Clin Infect Dis 2013; 57:781.
5. Katsanis GP, Spargo J, Ferraro MJ, et al. Detection of Klebsiella pneumoniae and Escherichia coli strains producing extended-spectrum beta-lactamases. J Clin Microbiol 1994; 32:691.
6. Wiener J, Quinn JP, Bradford PA, et al. Multiple antibiotic-resistant Klebsiella and Escherichia coli in nursing homes. JAMA 1999; 281:517.
7. Papanicolaou GA, Medeiros AA, Jacoby GA. Novel plasmid-mediated beta-lactamase (MIR-1) conferring resistance to oxyimino- and alpha-methoxy beta-lactams in clinical isolates of Klebsiella pneumoniae. Antimicrob Agents Chemother 1990; 34:2200.
8. Bratu S, Landman D, Haag R, et al. Rapid spread of carbapenem-resistant Klebsiella pneumoniae in New York City: a new threat to our antibiotic armamentarium. Arch Intern Med 2005; 165:1430.
9. Bratu S, Brooks S, Burney S, et al. Detection and spread of Escherichia coli possessing the plasmid-borne carbapenemase KPC-2 in Brooklyn, New York. Clin Infect Dis 2007; 44:972.
10. Kumarasamy KK, Toleman MA, Walsh TR, et al. Emergence of a new antibiotic resistance mechanism in India, Pakistan, and the UK: a molecular, biological, and epidemiological study. Lancet Infect Dis 2010; 10:597.

11. Asbel LE, Levison ME. Cephalosporins, carbapenems, and monobactams. Infect Dis Clin North Am 2000; 14:435.

12. FDA Drug Safety Communication: Cefepime and risk of seizure in patients not receiving dosage adjustments for kidney impairment, June 26, 2012. http://www.fda.gov/Drugs/DrugSafety/ucm309661.htm (Accessed on June 27, 2012).

13. Hooton TM. Clinical practice. Uncomplicated urinary tract infection. N Engl J Med 2012; 366:1028.

14. Gupta K, Trautner B. In the clinic. Urinary tract infection. Ann Intern Med 2012; 156:ITC3.

15. Hooton TM, Roberts PL, Cox ME, Stapleton AE. Voided midstream urine culture and acute cystitis in premenopausal women. N Engl J Med 2013; 369:1883.

16. Kahlmeter G. Prevalence and antimicrobial susceptibility of pathogens in uncomplicated cystitis in Europe. The ECO.SENS study. Int J Antimicrob Agents 2003; 22 Suppl 2:49.

17. Kahlmeter G, ECO.SENS. An international survey of the antimicrobial susceptibility of pathogens from uncomplicated urinary tract infections: the ECO.SENS Project. J Antimicrob Chemother 2003; 51:69.

18. Naber KG, Schito G, Botto H, et al. Surveillance study in Europe and Brazil on clinical aspects and Antimicrobial Resistance Epidemiology in Females with Cystitis (ARESC): implications for empiric therapy. Eur Urol 2008; 54:1164.

19. Zhanel GG, Hisanaga TL, Laing NM, et al. Antibiotic resistance in Escherichia coli outpatient urinary isolates: final results from the North American Urinary Tract Infection Collaborative Alliance (NAUTICA). Int J Antimicrob Agents 2006; 27:468.

20. Sanchez GV, Master RN, Karlowsky JA, Bordon JM. In vitro antimicrobial resistance of urinary Escherichia coli isolates among U.S. outpatients from 2000 to 2010. Antimicrob Agents Chemother 2012; 56:2181.

21. Swami SK, Liesinger JT, Shah N, et al. Incidence of antibiotic-resistant Escherichia coli bacteriuria according to age and location of onset: a population-based study from Olmsted County, Minnesota. Mayo Clin Proc 2012; 87:753.

22. Metlay JP, Fine MJ. Testing strategies in the initial management of patients with community-acquired pneumonia. Ann Intern Med 2003; 138:109.

23. Lim WS, van der Eerden MM, Laing R, et al. Defining community acquired pneumonia severity on presentation to hospital: an international derivation and validation study. Thorax 2003; 58:377.

24. Bauer TT, Ewig S, Marre R, et al. CRB-65 predicts death from community-acquired pneumonia. J Intern Med 2006; 260:93.

25. Marrie TJ, Shariatzadeh MR. Community-acquired pneumonia requiring admission to an intensive care unit: a descriptive study. Medicine (Baltimore) 2007; 86:103.

26. Marrie TJ, Poulin-Costello M, Beecroft MD, Herman-Gnjidic Z. Etiology of community-acquired pneumonia treated in an ambulatory setting. Respir Med 2005; 99:60.

27. Lim WS, Macfarlane JT, Boswell TC, et al. Study of community acquired pneumonia aetiology (SCAPA) in adults admitted to hospital: implications for management guidelines. Thorax 2001; 56:296.

28. Malcolm C, Marrie TJ. Antibiotic therapy for ambulatory patients with community-acquired pneumonia in an emergency department setting. Arch Intern Med 2003; 163:797.

29. Read RC. Evidence-based medicine: empiric antibiotic therapy in community-acquired pneumonia. J Infect 1999; 39:171.

30. File TM Jr, Niederman MS. Antimicrobial therapy of community-acquired pneumonia. Infect Dis Clin North Am 2004; 18:993.

31. Kuster SP, Rudnick W, Shigayeva A, et al. Previous antibiotic exposure and antimicrobial resistance in invasive pneumococcal disease: results from prospective surveillance. Clin Infect Dis 2014; 59:944.

32. Durack DT, Lukes AS, Bright DK. New criteria for diagnosis of infective endocarditis: utilization of specific echocardiographic findings. Duke Endocarditis Service. Am J Med 1994; 96:200.

33. Parker MT, Ball LC. Streptococci and aerococci associated with systemic infection in man. J Med Microbiol 1976; 9:275.

108

34. Anderson DJ, Murdoch DR, Sexton DJ, et al. Risk factors for infective endocarditis in patients with enterococcal bacteremia: a case-control study. Infection 2004; 32:72.

35. Li JS, Sexton DJ, Mick N, et al. Proposed modifications to the Duke criteria for the diagnosis of infective endocarditis. Clin Infect Dis 2000; 30:633.

36. Baddour LM, Wilson WR, Bayer AS, et al. Infective endocarditis: diagnosis, antimicrobial therapy, and management of complications: a statement for healthcare professionals from the Committee on Rheumatic Fever, Endocarditis, and Kawasaki Disease, Council on Cardiovascular Disease in the Young, and the Councils on Clinical Cardiology, Stroke, and Cardiovascular Surgery and Anesthesia, American Heart Association: endorsed by the Infectious Diseases Society of America. Circulation 2005; 111:e394.

37. Lindner JR, Case RA, Dent JM, et al. Diagnostic value of echocardiography in suspected endocarditis. An evaluation based on the pretest probability of disease. Circulation 1996; 93:730.

38. Nishimura RA, Otto CM, Bonow RO, et al. 2014 AHA/ACC guideline for the management of patients with valvular heart disease: a report of the American College of Cardiology/American Heart Association Task Force on Practice Guidelines. J Am Coll Cardiol 2014; 63:e57.

39. Shively BK, Gurule FT, Roldan CA, et al. Diagnostic value of transesophageal compared with transthoracic echocardiography in infective endocarditis. J Am Coll Cardiol 1991; 18:391.

40. Roghmann MC, Warner J, Mackowiak PA. The relationship between age and fever magnitude. Am J Med Sci 2001; 322:68.

41. Jurkat-Rott K, McCarthy T, Lehmann-Horn F. Genetics and pathogenesis of malignant hyperthermia. Muscle Nerve 2000; 23:4.

42. Karagianis JL, Phillips LC, Hogan KP, LeDrew KK. Clozapine-associated neuroleptic malignant syndrome: two new cases and a review of the literature. Ann Pharmacother 1999; 33:623.

43. Gurrera RJ. Sympathoadrenal hyperactivity and the etiology of neuroleptic malignant syndrome. Am J Psychiatry 1999; 156:169.

109

44. Bone RC. Gram-negative sepsis: a dilemma of modern medicine. Clin Microbiol Rev 1993; 6:57.

45. Dinarello CA. Infection, fever, and exogenous and endogenous pyrogens: some concepts have changed. J Endotoxin Res 2004; 10:201.

46. Schlievert PM, Shands KN, Dan BB, et al. Identification and characterization of an exotoxin from Staphylococcus aureus associated with toxic-shock syndrome. J Infect Dis 1981; 143:509.

47. Parsonnet J, Gillis ZA, Pier GB. Induction of interleukin-1 by strains of Staphylococcus aureus from patients with nonmenstrual toxic shock syndrome. J Infect Dis 1986; 154:55.

48. Tan T, Little P, Stokes T, Guideline Development Group. Antibiotic prescribing for self limiting respiratory tract infections in primary care: summary of NICE guidance. BMJ 2008; 337:a437.

49. King D, Mitchell B, Williams CP, Spurling GK. Saline nasal irrigation for acute upper respiratory tract infections. Cochrane Database Syst Rev 2015; 4:CD006821.

50. Louisiana Department of Health and Hospitals. http://new.dhh.louisiana.gov/index.cfm/newsroom/detail/2332 (Accessed on January 22, 2012).

51. Zalmanovici Trestioreanu A, Yaphe J. Intranasal steroids for acute sinusitis. Cochrane Database Syst Rev 2013; 12:CD005149.

52. Chow AW, Benninger MS, Brook I, et al. IDSA clinical practice guideline for acute bacterial rhinosinusitis in children and adults. Clin Infect Dis 2012; 54:e72.

53. Williamson IG, Rumsby K, Benge S, et al. Antibiotics and topical nasal steroid for treatment of acute maxillary sinusitis: a randomized controlled trial. JAMA 2007; 298:2487.

54. Bende M, Fukami M, Arfors KE, et al. Effect of oxymetazoline nose drops on acute sinusitis in the rabbit. Ann Otol Rhinol Laryngol 1996; 105:222.

55. Spector SL, Bernstein IL, Li JT, et al. Parameters for the diagnosis and management of sinusitis. J Allergy Clin Immunol 1998; 102:S107.

56. Rosenfeld RM, Piccirillo JF, Chandrasekhar SS, et al. Clinical practice guideline (update): adult sinusitis. Otolaryngol Head Neck Surg 2015; 152:S1.

110

57. Roth RP, Cantekin EI, Bluestone CD, et al. Nasal decongestant activity of pseudoephedrine. Ann Otol Rhinol Laryngol 1977; 86:235.

58. Melén I, Friberg B, Andréasson L, et al. Effects of phenylpropanolamine on ostial and nasal patency in patients treated for chronic maxillary sinusitis. Acta Otolaryngol 1986; 101:494.

59. Aust R, Drettner B, Falck B. Studies of the effect of peroral fenylpropanolamin on the functional size of the human maxillary ostium. Acta Otolaryngol 1979; 88:455.

60. MCLAURIN JW, SHIPMAN WF, ROSEDALE R Jr. Oral decongestants. A double blind comparison study of the effectiveness of four sympathomimetic drugs: objective and subjective. Laryngoscope 1961; 71:54.

61. Ziment I. Management of respiratory problems in the aged. J Am Geriatr Soc 1982; 30:S36.

62. Sandler RS. Epidemiology of irritable bowel syndrome in the United States. Gastroenterology 1990; 99:409.

63. Kay L. Prevalence, incidence and prognosis of gastrointestinal symptoms in a random sample of an elderly population. Age Ageing 1994; 23:146.

64. Fleischer AB Jr, Gardner EF, Feldman SR. Are patients' chief complaints generally specific to one organ system? Am J Manag Care 2001; 7:299.

65. Yamamoto W, Kono H, Maekawa M, Fukui T. The relationship between abdominal pain regions and specific diseases: an epidemiologic approach to clinical practice. J Epidemiol 1997; 7:27.

66. Heikkinen M, Pikkarainen P, Eskelinen M, Julkunen R. GPs' ability to diagnose dyspepsia based only on physical examination and patient history. Scand J Prim Health Care 2000; 18:99.

67. Thomson AB, Barkun AN, Armstrong D, et al. The prevalence of clinically significant endoscopic findings in primary care patients with uninvestigated dyspepsia: the Canadian Adult Dyspepsia Empiric Treatment - Prompt Endoscopy (CADET-PE) study. Aliment Pharmacol Ther 2003; 17:1481.

68. Böhner H, Yang Q, Franke C, et al. Simple data from history and physical examination help to exclude bowel obstruction and to avoid radiographic studies in patients with acute abdominal pain. Eur J Surg 1998; 164:777.

111

69. Eskelinen M, Ikonen J, Lipponen P. Usefulness of history-taking, physical examination and diagnostic scoring in acute renal colic. Eur Urol 1998; 34:467.

70. Trowbridge RL, Rutkowski NK, Shojania KG. Does this patient have acute cholecystitis? JAMA 2003; 289:80.

71. Thomas SH, Silen W, Cheema F, et al. Effects of morphine analgesia on diagnostic accuracy in Emergency Department patients with abdominal pain: a prospective, randomized trial. J Am Coll Surg 2003; 196:18.

72. Mahadevan M, Graff L. Prospective randomized study of analgesic use for ED patients with right lower quadrant abdominal pain. Am J Emerg Med 2000; 18:753.

73. Pace S, Burke TF. Intravenous morphine for early pain relief in patients with acute abdominal pain. Acad Emerg Med 1996; 3:1086.

74. Attard AR, Corlett MJ, Kidner NJ, et al. Safety of early pain relief for acute abdominal pain. BMJ 1992; 305:554.

75. Zoltie N, Cust MP. Analgesia in the acute abdomen. Ann R Coll Surg Engl 1986; 68:209.

76. Ranji SR, Goldman LE, Simel DL, Shojania KG. Do opiates affect the clinical evaluation of patients with acute abdominal pain? JAMA 2006; 296:1764.

77. Manterola C, Astudillo P, Losada H, et al. Analgesia in patients with acute abdominal pain. Cochrane Database Syst Rev 2007; :CD005660.

78. Jung PJ, Merrell RC. Acute abdomen. Gastroenterol Clin North Am 1988; 17:227.

79. Obuz F, Terzi C, Sökmen S, et al. The efficacy of helical CT in the diagnosis of small bowel obstruction. Eur J Radiol 2003; 48:299.

80. Schermer CR, Hanosh JJ, Davis M, Pitcher DE. Ogilvie's syndrome in the surgical patient: a new therapeutic modality. J Gastrointest Surg 1999; 3:173.

81. Laméris W, van Randen A, van Es HW, et al. Imaging strategies for detection of urgent conditions in patients with acute abdominal pain: diagnostic accuracy study. BMJ 2009; 338:b2431.

82. Cappell MS, Friedel D. Abdominal pain during pregnancy. Gastroenterol Clin North Am 2003; 32:1.

83. Morino M, Pellegrino L, Castagna E, et al. Acute nonspecific abdominal pain: A randomized, controlled trial comparing early laparoscopy versus clinical observation. Ann Surg 2006; 244:881.

112

84. Romagnuolo J, Bardou M, Rahme E, et al. Magnetic resonance cholangiopancreatography: a meta-analysis of test performance in suspected biliary disease. Ann Intern Med 2003; 139:547.

85. Bytzer P, Hansen JM, Havelund T, et al. Predicting endoscopic diagnosis in the dyspeptic patient: the value of clinical judgement. Eur J Gastroenterol Hepatol 1996; 8:359.

86. Timmons S, Liston R, Moriarty KJ. Functional dyspepsia: motor abnormalities, sensory dysfunction, and therapeutic options. Am J Gastroenterol 2004; 99:739.

87. Lewin van den Broek NT, Numans ME, Buskens E, et al. A randomised controlled trial of four management strategies for dyspepsia: relationships between symptom subgroups and strategy outcome. Br J Gen Pract 2001; 51:619.

88. Yadav D, Agarwal N, Pitchumoni CS. A critical evaluation of laboratory tests in acute pancreatitis. Am J Gastroenterol 2002; 97:1309.

89. Domingo P, Mancebo J, Blanch L, et al. Fever in adult patients with acute bacterial meningitis. J Infect Dis 1988; 158:496.

90. Thomas KE, Hasbun R, Jekel J, Quagliarello VJ. The diagnostic accuracy of Kernig's sign, Brudzinski's sign, and nuchal rigidity in adults with suspected meningitis. Clin Infect Dis 2002; 35:46.

91. Choi C. Bacterial meningitis in aging adults. Clin Infect Dis 2001; 33:1380.

92. Attia J, Hatala R, Cook DJ, Wong JG. The rational clinical examination. Does this adult patient have acute meningitis? JAMA 1999; 282:175.

93. Schut ES, Lucas MJ, Brouwer MC, et al. Cerebral infarction in adults with bacterial meningitis. Neurocrit Care 2012; 16:421.

94. Zoons E, Weisfelt M, de Gans J, et al. Seizures in adults with bacterial meningitis. Neurology 2008; 70:2109.

95. Mylonakis E, Hohmann EL, Calderwood SB. Central nervous system infection with Listeria monocytogenes. 33 years' experience at a general hospital and review of 776 episodes from the literature. Medicine (Baltimore) 1998; 77:313.

96. Brouwer MC, van de Beek D, Heckenberg SG, et al. Community-acquired Listeria monocytogenes meningitis in adults. Clin Infect Dis 2006; 43:1233.

97. Heckenberg SG, de Gans J, Brouwer MC, et al. Clinical features, outcome, and meningococcal genotype in 258 adults with meningococcal meningitis: a prospective cohort study. Medicine (Baltimore) 2008; 87:185.

98. Pace D, Pollard AJ. Meningococcal disease: clinical presentation and sequelae. Vaccine 2012; 30 Suppl 2:B3.

99. Weisfelt M, van de Beek D, Spanjaard L, de Gans J. Arthritis in adults with community-acquired bacterial meningitis: a prospective cohort study. BMC Infect Dis 2006; 6:64.

100. Uchihara T, Tsukagoshi H. Jolt accentuation of headache: the most sensitive sign of CSF pleocytosis. Headache 1991; 31:167.

101. Nakao JH, Jafri FN, Shah K, Newman DH. Jolt accentuation of headache and other clinical signs: poor predictors of meningitis in adults. Am J Emerg Med 2014; 32:24.

102. Tamune H, Takeya H, Suzuki W, et al. Absence of jolt accentuation of headache cannot accurately rule out meningitis in adults. Am J Emerg Med 2013; 31:1601.

103. Kaplan SL. Clinical presentations, diagnosis, and prognostic factors of bacterial meningitis. Infect Dis Clin North Am 1999; 13:579.

104. Kornelisse RF, Westerbeek CM, Spoor AB, et al. Pneumococcal meningitis in children: prognostic indicators and outcome. Clin Infect Dis 1995; 21:1390.

105. Brouwer MC, van de Beek D, Heckenberg SG, et al. Hyponatraemia in adults with community-acquired bacterial meningitis. QJM 2007; 100:37.

106. Geiseler PJ, Nelson KE, Levin S, et al. Community-acquired purulent meningitis: a review of 1,316 cases during the antibiotic era, 1954-1976. Rev Infect Dis 1980; 2:725.

107. Talan DA, Hoffman JR, Yoshikawa TT, Overturf GD. Role of empiric parenteral antibiotics prior to lumbar puncture in suspected bacterial meningitis: state of the art. Rev Infect Dis 1988; 10:365.

108. Kanegaye JT, Soliemanzadeh P, Bradley JS. Lumbar puncture in pediatric bacterial meningitis: defining the time interval for recovery of cerebrospinal fluid pathogens after parenteral antibiotic pretreatment. Pediatrics 2001; 108:1169.

109. Brouwer MC, Thwaites GE, Tunkel AR, van de Beek D. Dilemmas in the diagnosis of acute community-acquired bacterial meningitis. Lancet 2012; 380:1684.

110. Hasbun R, Abrahams J, Jekel J, Quagliarello VJ. Computed tomography of the head before lumbar puncture in adults with suspected meningitis. N Engl J Med 2001; 345:1727.

111. Gopal AK, Whitehouse JD, Simel DL, Corey GR. Cranial computed tomography before lumbar puncture: a prospective clinical evaluation. Arch Intern Med 1999; 159:2681.

112. Tunkel AR, Hartman BJ, Kaplan SL, et al. Practice guidelines for the management of bacterial meningitis. Clin Infect Dis 2004; 39:1267.

113. Joffe AR. Lumbar puncture and brain herniation in acute bacterial meningitis: a review. J Intensive Care Med 2007; 22:194.

114. Glimåker M, Johansson B, Grindborg Ö, et al. Adult bacterial meningitis: earlier treatment and improved outcome following guideline revision promoting prompt lumbar puncture. Clin Infect Dis 2015; 60:1162.

115. Blazer S, Berant M, Alon U. Bacterial meningitis. Effect of antibiotic treatment on cerebrospinal fluid. Am J Clin Pathol 1983; 80:386.

116. Spanos A, Harrell FE Jr, Durack DT. Differential diagnosis of acute meningitis. An analysis of the predictive value of initial observations. JAMA 1989; 262:2700.

117. Huy NT, Thao NT, Diep DT, et al. Cerebrospinal fluid lactate concentration to distinguish bacterial from aseptic meningitis: a systemic review and meta-analysis. Crit Care 2010; 14:R240.

118. Cox NH. Palpation of the skin--an important issue. J R Soc Med 2006; 99:598.

119. Petit A, Tailor A. Skin Semiology and Grading Scales. In: Ethnic Dermatology - Principles and Practice, Dadzie OE, Petit A, Alexis AF (Eds), Wiley-Blackwell, Oxford, UK 2013.

120. Al-Dabagh A, Davis SA, McMichael AJ, Feldman SR. Rosacea in skin of color: not a rare diagnosis. Dermatol Online J 2014; 20.

121. Kundu RV, Patterson S. Dermatologic conditions in skin of color: part II. Disorders occurring predominately in skin of color. Am Fam Physician 2013; 87:859.

122. Argenziano G, Soyer HP. Dermoscopy of pigmented skin lesions--a valuable tool for early diagnosis of melanoma. Lancet Oncol 2001; 2:443.

123. Haliasos HC, Zalaudek I, Malvehy J, et al. Dermoscopy of benign and malignant neoplasms in the pediatric population. Semin Cutan Med Surg 2010; 29:218.
124. Argenziano G, Puig S, Zalaudek I, et al. Dermoscopy improves accuracy of primary care physicians to triage lesions suggestive of skin cancer. J Clin Oncol 2006; 24:1877.

Made in the USA
Lexington, KY
29 September 2015